DR. HUSTLE

9 Core Principles to Help You Build a Thriving Practice in Today's Competitive, Constantly Changing Healthcare Market

Kevin Kruse, M.D.

ISBN-13: 978-0-578-78774-9

Printed in the U.S.A.

Editing: Daria Anne DiGiovanni, Jodi Hinkle
Cover Design: Zeljka Kojic

❖ Table of Contents

Dedication

To my beautiful wife Stephanie, for her love and support,
and for allowing me to chase my dreams.

Introduction

Redefining "Hustle."

It happened in my third year of residency, during a visit to my hometown. I met up with an orthopedic surgeon I had known since high school, the same guy who had scoped my knee when I played football in college. I asked for his advice as to securing a job in the Dallas metro area and informed him I would be doing a fellowship in both shoulder and hand surgery.

From an orthopedic standpoint, the area appeared to be saturated and I was concerned about my ability to carve out a busy practice in that environment. I will never forget what he told me. "Kevin, you could go there and make a killing, but you have got to be willing to hustle."

Hustle.

It surprised me a little to hear a surgeon use that word to describe the attitude I would have to take to build a thriving practice in a highly competitive environment. Never in my life had I thought of comparing a busy orthopedic surgeon to a hustler. To me, a hustler was someone who made shady deals in pool halls and pawn shops – not a professional who had dedicated his life to the practice of medicine and sworn a Hippocratic Oath. For reasons that will become clear, I have since come to love that word.

According to the dictionary definition, a hustler is "an aggressively enterprising person." These days, when I think of the word, "hustler," I consider the ten thousand essential elements for building a busy, successful orthopedic practice. As I have learned, it is not just about working hard but working *smart*. It is about choosing where to focus most of your energy…and where not to. Hustlers know how to play the game and, more importantly, how to win it.

So, why did I choose a career in medicine and a specialty in orthopedics? It all begins with my father, a successful physician in his own right. Growing up in Carmel, Indiana, a suburb of Indianapolis, I saw the admiration people felt for him, and it instilled a sense of pride in me. I witnessed his dedication to his profession and his patients, and, over and over, I heard people tell me how much he had helped them. I felt proud to have a dad who was a doctor.

I also excelled in school, particularly when I applied myself to subjects like biology and to the art of test-taking, which expanded my desire to follow in my father's footsteps. My participation in sports further nurtured my interest in medicine. Eventually, I selected football as my main sport and walked onto the football team at Indiana University. The life lessons I learned from playing this hard-hitting game helped to shape the person I am today.

As a high school and college football player, you must apply the discipline to train, handle injuries, cooperate with the other players on your team, and – most importantly – handle failures. When you are a walk-on player in college, you do not get a lot of respect. They treat you roughly. Throughout my football years, I sustained multiple injuries that required surgery. Having to play with injuries and cope with the pain toughened me up quite a bit and helped me discover how the world truly works. I learned that, despite your most diligent efforts, the endeavor itself can fail. Notwithstanding my hard work, I never achieved my goal of earning a scholarship, nor did our team accomplish our goal of winning. We prevailed in few games.

Some people might look at these experiences and remark, "Wow, you sustained a bunch of injuries, you never got your scholarship, and your team lost more games than they won. What a massive failure on multiple levels!" Perhaps on the surface, this would be an accurate observation, but the injuries I suffered inspired me to become an orthopedic surgeon, which turned out to be a rewarding, wonderful career. The moral of the story is that you can work your butt off to attain a specific goal and still not reach it; however, if you can find the lessons, forge greater discipline, and develop meaningful relationships as a result of the experience, you can apply them to achieve the success you envision.

In my experience, the mental toughness and time management skills I developed as a Division 1 student athlete who managed a difficult pre-med curriculum molded me as a human being and set the foundation for the career I enjoy today. I am grateful I took these risks at a young age because it taught me how to take on bigger risks and lay everything on the line – win or lose. Take it from me: your temporary failures will aid you in the accomplishment of long-term successes.

By the time I got accepted into Indiana University Medical School, I had already suffered several orthopedic injuries, solidifying my decision to become an orthopedic surgeon. During my med school years, I sustained many more, followed by another one in residency. In all, I had a total of five orthopedic surgeries throughout my life.

Once I selected my speciality, my work was just beginning. To get into a competitive subspecialty like orthopedics, I had to study hard to make it into the top 10- to- 15 percent of my medical school class – no easy feat since med school students are not exactly slouches. Fortunately, in my first year of medical school, one of the best things that has ever happened to me took place: I met my wife, Stephanie.

She and I first laid eyes on each other at a hog roast, given by a friend of mine during a party weekend at Indiana University. I was coming back for my first year of medical school and she had just returned from L.A., having decided to give up her career in pop music and acting to return to her hometown of Indianapolis. As the story goes, we started dating, one thing led to another, and eventually we got married.

After med school, I matched in a residency program in Greenville, South Carolina, a place where neither of us had roots. I had interviewed for 18 programs and had chosen Denver Colorado as my first preference, just because I thought it sounded like an awesome place to live. However, when I went to Greenville for my interview, I discovered their program was amazing. From the outset, the thing that struck me the most was how happy all the residents seemed; none of them appeared burned out or beat down.

On the contrary, they seemed thrilled to be there and felt as if they received excellent training. The fact that I could play golf year-round was another plus because golf is one of my passions. I marked Greenville as my second choice, even though my gut told me I was going to end up there. And when I opened my envelope on Match Day, my instincts were proven correct: we were indeed heading to Greenville.

Matching in a residency is a huge decision because it is five years of your life…and yet, it also depends on the randomness of the universe and the multitude of factors that determine where you get selected. I was lucky to be placed at my second choice, where we spent an amazing five years. Stephanie and I got married as soon as we moved to Greenville and had our first child about a year later – much sooner than we had anticipated. In my third year of residency, we had our second child.

We bought a cute little house on a charming street, where we threw countless parties, surrounded by tons of friends. It sounds strange; most people talk about residency as being a huge beatdown, but mine was fantastic. Early on, they pushed us to the limit, and worked us hard, but in the later years in was much more of a team effort. We took our licks early and enjoyed a lighter workload later. I learned how to operate and become an excellent surgeon in a fulfilling environment. Now, I look back on those five years as some of the best times of my life.

Like so many experiences before and after, my Greenville residency made an enormous impact on my life and career. In my second year of residency, I chose the orthopedic subspecialty of shoulder and elbow – partly because I had surgery on my own shoulder and elbow, and partly because I loved the anatomy of the upper extremity and treating all the pathologies that occur within it. I chose a fellowship in Pittsburgh that technically fell under the hand fellowship match but still allowed me to perform quite a bit of complex elbow and hand surgery.

After Pittsburgh, at the recommendation of Dr. Richard Hawkins in Greenville – a world renowned shoulder surgeon, I opted to go to Lyon France to complete an international fellowship with Dr. Gilles Walsh. There was just one problem: I had not figured out how to pay for it, since it was not a paid fellowship. I had to cover my expenses out of my own pocket – which was crazy, since I had no savings, nor did I have a job. To earn some money, I returned to South Carolina to do a month of locum tenens. The roughly $35,000 I made was enough to get us to France and complete most of my fellowship.

In August of 2015, my wife and two kids joined me on this new adventure, where we spent four months immersing ourselves in the French culture. Working with Dr. Walsh and his team of shoulder surgeons provided the last incredible step in my training. Having distilled my interest in orthopedics down to the upper extremity, shoulder, and hand, my fellowship with Dr. Walsh enabled me to hone my craft and truly learn how to perform shoulder surgery.

Prior to that, I thought I knew most of what I needed to know to start a practice but studying with Dr. Walsh opened my mind and molded the practice I have today. Because it was highly specialized and the last step in my journey before embarking upon my practice, it continues to influence the way I think about, treat, and operate on shoulders. Dr. Walsh is a master surgeon and an amazing human being. I cannot praise him enough.

Upon returning to the United States, Stephanie and I thought it would be an excellent idea to open my job search to various groups across the entire country. During our time in Pittsburgh, her family had moved out of the Indianapolis area – which was a huge blessing because it gave me the freedom to choose a job and a practice that felt like the right fit for me. After an exhausting and stressful 20 interviews with various groups, I was panicking about getting hired. That is when I called a practice in Dallas that had just lost their phenomenal upper extremity surgeon. I knew of him because he had trained many of the guys with whom I spent my residency. It was a blessing because they were eager to replace him.

As a family, we decided to move to Dallas, where we had no ties and no extended family. We had not even spent any significant time there but had heard from others who had lived there that it was a great place to put down roots. We moved to the Park Cities, an upscale, affluent area within the city limits that boasts an excellent school system and a high standard of living. Our family has never been happier.

An ultra-competitive orthopedic environment, Dallas is home to many world-renowned surgeons, which meant that for me to survive, I had to assume the mentality of a hustler every single day. Part of that involved regular brainstorming sessions with my partner, Brett Raynor, centered on how to build busy orthopedic practices. After countless meetings and five years in practice, I am proud to tell you that both of us have achieved and surpassed many of our goals. As someone who has always loved the idea of using objective measurements to make improvements, it is a thrill for me to review the financial books every month at our practice. At the end of the year last year, the numbers revealed that Raynor and I were the highest collectors in the group – quite a feat for two young doctors whose partners have practiced in Dallas for over 30 years!

I do not have to explain the significance of this accomplishment to a practicing surgeon. If you are just beginning your surgical practice, you have probably heard these words of wisdom from your more seasoned colleagues: "Work hard, treat people like gold, and you will get busy." While this is sage advice, I know from experience that developing a busy practice entails so much more.

Doesn't every orthopedic surgeon treat people well and do their best work? Is there any surgeon in practice who believes they can treat their patients poorly, perform subpar surgeries, and enjoy a thriving career?

I am reasonably certain that every young surgeon embarking upon their practice already understands that at a bare minimum, they must relate well to their patients and perform excellent surgery. Keep in mind that your colleagues who have been in practice for a decade or more are in a much different place. Presumably, they have already built a successful practice, so it only makes sense to seek their advice. That is the conventional wisdom in life: to learn from others who have already achieved the goals you have set for yourself. There is no substitute for experience, and I encourage you to heed their advice…with an important caveat. Today's healthcare market is rapidly changing and evolving. The principles that worked well for your seasoned colleagues back in the day may not work for you now.

There are core principles you can apply and learn to accelerate the growth of your busy practice. Based on Raynor's and my experience, this book lays out our blueprint and explains all the "little" things we have learned over the past four years on the way to building a thriving practice in an ultra competitive city. The more I thought about what we had accomplished, the more I realized we could help young doctors coming into practice who might benefit from the lessons we have learned. Remember, there is no teacher greater than experience. This book is my attempt to tell the story of how two newbie surgeons grinded out bustling practices in an intensely competitive metro area. It is my hope that it guides you in understanding the actions we took and motivates you to attain the practice you have been dreaming of.

Chapter 1

Analyze Your Billing and Coding

When I was a fourth-year resident, I attended a fellows' course for shoulder arthroplasty. At the end, one of the surgeons spoke to the fellows about practice management, using a real-life story to illustrate his point. For over a year and a half, a biller for a total joint surgeon in his group had neglected to include the modifier for bilateral total knees. Once they discovered the errors and attempted to resubmit to the insurance company, it was too late. The insurance company informed them that they were past the point of no return and refused to reimburse them for services rendered.

Because of one simple error, the surgeon lost over *$150,000* in collections.

That story motivated me to audit my codes every single month. At month's end, I sit down with my biller and review every CPT code I submitted for surgery. I take note of what the insurance company paid and ensure that all the surgeries were accurately coded. That said, I am the one who submits the codes to my biller. You would think this should be a seamless process with few, if any, mistakes, but I always find some. It does not matter how competent your biller is, they are human, and all humans make mistakes. When it comes to CPT codes, these human errors can cost you thousands of dollars a month.

Accurate billing and coding can make or break your practice – which is why it amazes me that surgeons tend to neglect this vital aspect of their business. Some of the easiest money you will ever make (or lose) will be contingent upon your understanding and monitoring of your billing and coding. Yet many physicians overlook this crucial part of their income stream and delegate it to someone else. Yes, you must employ a full-time biller that either works in your office or offsite. And yes, you must monitor and audit the billing. Why? Because no one understands the coding and the level surgery of surgery you perform…and they never will. Only you know what you did in the operating room; therefore, you are the only one who has the knowledge to accurately code what you did in surgery and in the clinic.

When you consider how hard we work for the money we make, this is a miniscule amount of time – we're talking about 20 to 30 minutes a month to sit down and make sure all the codes were submitted properly. Again, your biller will get it right 95 percent of the time. But that five percent can cost you quite a bit.

I put this principle into practice by reviewing the last three months to make sure everything gets paid and to determine whether the insurance company rejected one of our claims or not. In the case of a rejection, we write an appropriate letter, mainly to confirm the codes are correct for the surgeries performed. In this process, I almost always catch a few small errors that add up to a massive amount of money over the course of a year – to the tune of tens of thousands of dollars.

As the surgeon, I advise you to code all your surgeries because you understand the CPT codes better than anybody. Of course, if you have a specific question about coding, ask your billing expert or visit one of the coding websites to make sure you are billing correctly. You never want to code for more or less than what you do.

Surgeons tend to rely on billers too much. I cannot stress enough how important it is to make sure you submit your CPT codes for every surgery you perform. Plan a time every month to meet with your biller in person – or if they work offsite, schedule a phone or ZOOM call – for the purpose of examining every single surgery you performed, confirming the codes are correct, and determining whether or not the insurance company pays you for your completed cases.

It is also nice to know how much money you earn for your surgeries. As with any other business, a practicing surgeon should track how much money they generate for each case. To succeed, you must cultivate a thorough understanding of the ins and outs of your mini business within the practice.

One of the best ways to support these efforts is to open the CPT coding book and read the sections that explain the various codes for your most common surgeries. Often, you will discover you have been doing work that you are not submitting codes for. By understanding the language in the coding books as they relate to the surgeries you perform, you can code all your cases properly. You simply cannot accomplish this if you do not know a code exists, as I learned from my own experience.

One day, as I was discussing total knees with a friend of mine, I explained that I use a computer navigation program for my total shoulders. I did not even know that code existed. I had failed to review the latest coding books. My friend showed me the code he had been using for total knees, and now I use the same code for my shoulders. Granted, it is a small reimbursement, but considering I perform 125 of these procedures a year, it adds up significantly. This is yet another example of why billing and coding is vital.

AUDIT YOUR CLINIC

Another highly overlooked portion of an orthopedic surgeon's income is the work they do in clinic. Audit your clinic to ensure you are receiving the correct payments for services rendered. Furthermore, understand the rules between level 3 and level 4 visits – what distinguishes an established patient from a non-established patient. Two- to- three times a year, I audit my clinic collections and occasionally find big discrepancies. For example, after I had completed 20 to 30 ultrasound-guided injections of the suprascapular nerve, I asked my biller what we were collecting on them because I could not find the code in our system. It turned out that while the code was in our EMR, it was not the coding software linked to it; therefore, she had not been receiving the code. Together, we reviewed and billed all the codes, which amounted to several thousands in collections. If I had not kept a close eye on the situation, I could have easily missed it.

It is critical that you understand the rules and code accurately. *You do not want to leave money on the table.* It is all about being efficient and getting paid for your excellent work.

Do not be lazy about this.

You are costing yourself thousands of dollars if you do not learn to code.

CHAPTER 1 PRESCRIPTIONS FOR A HEALTHY PRACTICE

❖ Code your own surgeries and review your collections monthly.

❖ Employ a full-time biller.

❖ Code efficiently and appropriately.

QUESTIONS TO CONSIDER...REMEMBER, ACCURATE BILLING AND CODING CAN MAKE OR BREAK YOUR PRACTICE

1. How do I audit my **surgical codes** and collections every month to ensure I receive the maximum payment possible?

_____
_____
_____
_____
_____
_____
_____

2. How do I audit my **clinic** codes to make sure I am collecting appropriately for the work I do?

_____
_____
_____
_____
_____
_____
_____

3. What process have I put in place to provide open lines of communication between my biller and me?

_____

_____

_____

_____

_____

_____

_____

4. When was the last time I read the CPT coding books for the common surgeries I perform? Do I know the average reimbursements for the surgeries I perform by all my common payers? Do I understand which codes are bundled and which are not?

_____

_____

_____

_____

_____

_____

_____

Chapter 2

Establish Clinic Efficiency

One of my friends and colleagues is an extremely busy shoulder specialist who, along with his two physician assistants, sees over two-hundred patients a week in his office – an impressive accomplishment for a 40-year-old guy, eight years into his practice. In addition, he publishes ten- to- fifteen peer-reviewed papers every year and maintains a hectic travel schedule to teach and speak at conferences about once a month. He balances his thriving career with a personal life that includes a spouse and children.

Given his accomplishments, I asked him to share his approaches to work and family. How does he achieve such a high level of professional and personal proficiency? "First," he explained, "make it a daily habit to ask yourself, 'What can I do to be more efficient in my clinic?' Second, pose the same question to your staff, MA, PA, X-ray tech, and the front desk."

However, there is a caveat: it is not simply about efficiency, it is also about maintaining quality. You cannot focus solely shaving down time unless you want to risk your entire career. Sure, you could walk into an examining room and inform your patient that they have bad arthritis, need a joint replacement, and will be out in 30 seconds. While it may be incredibly efficient, my guess is you will not be doing much surgery if you take this approach. On the flip side, you cannot spend over an hour in an examining room with every patient. The key is to strike the right balance of maximum efficiency and high-quality care.

Your level of efficiency makes little difference if you do not have any patients to treat – or if your existing patients feel they do not get enough time with you, you do not listen to them, or they do not receive good care, whatever the reason. Therefore, your goal is to increase your efficiency while upholding high-quality standards. That is the objective of the Dr. Hustle game. To win it, you must pose multiple questions to yourself on a continual basis:

➤ How do I improve the overall patient experience, from the moment they walk through my office doors, undergo surgery, and complete their postoperative care?

➤ How do I improve the interactions with my front desk?

➤ How do I improve the interactions with my MA, X-ray techs, surgery schedulers, surgery center/hospital?

➤ How can I improve the communication between the patient and me to help them understand their forthcoming operation, the preoperative course, the early postoperative course, the late postoperative course, and all the potential issues that may arise?

➤ How can I clearly explain to my patient what type of physical therapy is required, what they can and cannot do, when they should expect to go back to work (depending on the nature of their job), and what their limitations are?

On a superficial level, most patients want to understand why you are doing what you are doing. Your role as the professional is to help them understand the procedure without bogging them down in technicalities. Can you keep it simple enough to enable them to comprehend the course of treatment without glossing over too many details?

Do your best to intuit the kind of patient you are dealing with. Is it someone who wants a ton of intricate detail – for example, an engineer who wants to the know the percent concentration of certain metals in the alloys of the implant – or someone who simply wants a general under-standing because they came to see you at the recommendation of a friend, and therefore, trust in your integrity and ability?

Keep in mind, this is a team game: the patient's experience is not just with you, but with every single person with whom they come into contact. That includes your scheduler, MA, nurses, technicians, PA — in essence everyone they interact with is an extension of you and your practice, which is why everyone on your staff must be involved in those questions.

Empower your team to brainstorm creative solutions. Encourage them to offer their input. You might think you have an excellent idea, only to have it shot down by your MA or PA for valid reasons. Perhaps it could harm another aspect of your practice. Maybe your patients might not like the proposal. Be willing to listen and respond to criticism. Remember, your practice is a complex system that is the summation of many smaller systems. The more complex a system, the more easily a small change in one place can negatively impact something else. Often what may seem to be a trivial change that makes total sense to you will impair something or someone else in a way that you had never conceived.

Furthermore, your team may have an abundance of ideas you had never even thought of with respect to issues you do not even think about. That is why it is vital to keep your staff involved. It is not just about you telling them what to do; it is about everybody putting their heads together and working synergistically toward a shared goal.

CHAPTER 2 PRESCRIPTIONS FOR A HEALTHY PRACTICE

❖ Do not be afraid to ask all the questions.

❖ Most patients want to know on a basic level what you will be doing to treat/solve their medical problem.

❖ The patient's overall experience involves more than just you.

QUESTIONS TO CONSIDER...REMEMBER, QUALITY MUST ACCOMPANY EFFICIENCY

1. How can I become more efficient in my clinic without sacrificing quality?

_____

_____

_____

_____

_____

_____

_____

_____

2. Do I sit down with my staff and regularly discuss what we can do as a team to be more efficient in clinic?

_____

_____

_____

_____

_____

_____

_____

_____

3. How do I improve the overall patient experience from start to finish?

_____

_____

_____

_____

_____

_____

_____

4. What systems can we put in place that help achieve both goals?

_____

_____

_____

_____

_____

_____

_____

5. How do we measure our progress?

_____

_____

_____

_____

_____

_____

_____

Chapter 3

Know What to Do When Things Get Rough in the OR

You are going to encounter difficult cases. It is a requirement for being an excellent orthopedic surgeon. Often, cases you did not anticipate would be a challenge can pose the most demanding problems. In this chapter, I will share a few tips I picked up from my mentors over the years, in addition to the lessons I have learned being out in practice.

When you first begin your practice and confront an unusually difficult case, one that will stretch your abilities, it is an excellent idea to invite a second orthopedic surgeon to join you – whether it is a young surgeon close to your age and skill level, or an older, more seasoned and adept surgeon. Either way, a second set of skilled hands and critical eyes in the OR ensures that the case will unfold much more smoothly almost all the time.

How do I know? During my first few years of practice I did this whenever I had a revision shoulder arthroplasty case, with excellent results. Aside from the benefit of the other surgeon's knowledge and expertise, it helps to have a confidante in the OR when things get rough, so you can calm and reassure each other that everything is going to be okay. For taxing cases, be sure to have a second orthopedist scrubbing with you – especially during your first year or two in practice.

When things start to go awry in the operating room, I cannot stress enough how important it is to keep your head and your cool. Many times, you will experience overpowering emotions when the procedure is not going well: you feel for the patient; you feel for yourself; and you feel for the staff, as if you are causing a delay for them. All these thoughts and emotions compound your stress, making it harder to maintain your composure and focus.

However, you must stay calm (or at least appear that way). You are the captain of the ship and the buck stops with you. The people watching you in the operating room can sense how the operation is going by your emotions and body language. Regardless of the difficulty, if you portray a sense of confidence and control, everyone in the room will respond in kind. They will remain calm, with the understanding that their work continues until the operation is completed.

By contrast, when you start to get flustered, it makes them nervous and more likely to make mistakes – thereby adding to your frustration. No matter how horrible your internal assessment of the situation, always exude confidence and control, even if you feel like running out of the room as you think to yourself, "What have I gotten myself into? This is brutal!"

Often, when it appears an operation is not going well, it helps to pause for ten- to- fifteen seconds to take a few deep breaths and clear your mind. I do this while I irrigate the wound. Next time you face a stressful situation in the OR, grab some irrigation and irrigate the wound thoroughly for a good 20- to- 30 seconds. As you do, inhale and exhale, quiet your mind, and observe as the water flows in and out of the incision. I refer to it as a "reset," because often the answers will just come to you. Our subconscious mind is powerful, but when we give in to stress, we block its ability to guide us. Just pretend that all that normal saline is washing the troubles away.

When you allow stress to overwhelm you as you operate on a patient, your mind cannot think clearly. Your motions and motor functions are not as skilled. To solve the problem, you must calm your brain and mind and get the job done. It only impedes your ability to perform a successful operation if you get upset, scream, yell, throw things, and create an atmosphere of dread and fear in the OR.

Let me reiterate, you must remain calm all the time.

Surgery is a lot like golf. When you play well, you think it is easy and fun. You wonder, "How the hell did I ever struggle at this game?" In that moment, you are in total control of your swing and the ball is doing exactly what you want it to. Then, all the sudden, you hook one into the trees. Next, you attempt a miracle shot out of the trees…but the ball hits a branch before it ricochets into a worse lie than you started with! You finally take your medicine and chip out to make your double or triple bogey. As you step up to the next tee, you are still berating yourself for being stupid for trying that shot. "You idiot," you think, "you had such a good round going!"

You feel the tension rising in your arms, chest, and hands. On the next swing off the tee, your preoccupation with that damn last pull hook causes you to block one a mile right out of bounds.

The key to success, whether as a golfer or a surgeon, is to recognize when things are starting to go off track. From there, take a deep breath, step back, and analyze what just happened, without allowing your emotions to affect your thinking and actions. You do not compound one mistake with another. The best golfers follow up double bogeys with birdies; the best surgeons make mistakes but quickly recognize and fix them. They move on without succumbing to their emotions. Now, part of the reason skilled golfers can do this is because they have the confidence of knowing they have done it before. They can withdraw from their memory bank all the similar situations they have confronted before, along with how they got back on track.

It is no different as a surgeon. You must accept that things will go wrong, and you will have to problem-solve one way or another. When you handle a situation well, save it in your hard drive so that the next time it happens, you can tap into the memory. All the sudden, it is no big deal. You can say to yourself. "I have made this mistake before. Yes, it sucks, and I am pissed, but I know exactly how to fix it!"

I recall an incident during one of my fellowships when we were doing a reverse shoulder with someone I regard as the best surgeon in the entire world. As he reduced the shoulder, it was tight. In the next moment, we heard, "*Crack*!" As the surgeon pulled out the retractor and examined the humerus, he muttered a few curse words. We all looked at each other in disbelief: *this surgeon is the best in the world, he cannot possibly make mistakes!*

Well, I soon realized the reason why he is the best surgeon in the world is because he handles mistakes well – not because he never makes them. After quickly getting his anger out of his system (literally one curse word) he asked for the cable and cement in a calm voice. He pulled out the stem and placed the cables around the fracture. Then he cemented in a new stem and reduced it. The entire process added no more than fifteen minutes to the case. In fact, if you had not observed closely, you would have hardly noticed that anything went wrong at all. It became clear to me that this was not his first time: he had faced this situation before and he knew exactly what to do. Even the best surgeons in the world confront mistakes and problems during surgery. It is the way they deal with them that makes them special.

OVERESTIMATE YOUR ALLOTTED TIME FOR CASES

When you first start in practice, book your cases for much longer than they take. Why? Your staff does not really understand that although it is a total knee, it is an exceptionally difficult total knee. It does not matter that one of your senior doctors does a total knee in thirty minutes. The office staff will notice if you schedule cases for five- to- 10 minutes that consistently take 30- to- 40 minutes, of if you schedule cases for 45 minutes- to- an hour that take several hours. If you inform them up front that a case will take four hours, and it takes four hours, that is okay. I recommend always giving yourself a little bit of time. The patient goes into it the appointment expecting it to take whatever amount of time you booked it for. If you take less time than scheduled, you are a good surgeon. If you take more time than scheduled, you are a bad surgeon. The perception is as simple as that.

It does not matter if the surgery unfolded smoothly, or the degree of difficulty involved. In their mind, if you work faster than you anticipated, you are better than you thought. If you work slower than the allotted time, you are worse than you thought. Therefore, book your cases for more time than you expect them to take on the front.

That said, you do not need to book a carpal tunnel release for four hours. Give yourself some wiggle room for cases without overdoing it. Straightforward cases can demand much more time than you estimate, for various reasons, such as a pin that breaks, or someone handing you the wrong instrument or screw. There are always things that can go wrong in the operating room, so allow yourself more time than you think you need.

Once again, I cannot stress enough the importance of exuding a steady sense of calm and control in the OR. Not only will it help you perform up to your best standards, it will help you to develop a good reputation. You do not want to be known as the young surgeon who spazzes out all the time in the OR, causes more stress, and creates an unpleasant work environment. Your team will adore you if you treat them with respect and make surgery enjoyable. No, you do not have to be chummy and joke around with everybody all the time. So long as you are cordial, calm, controlled, and smooth, they will love you.

What can you expect in return? The best technicians will want to work with you and give you their best because they respect you. Conversely, if your cases always take much longer than planned and every other case you do turns into an absolute shitshow, it will drag them down. They will not give you their best performance because they are stressed out and hate working with you. Remember this is a team game.

Picture yourself as a resident.

If your attending had an obnoxious personality and you couldn't stand them, did they get the best out of you? Did you prepare for and give every case one hundred percent? By contrast, if you felt respect and admiration for an attending, even when dealing with a case you did not particularly like, you remained focused. You relaxed. You had fun. And you performed at your highest level. Do not underestimate the importance of a positive attitude in the operating room. Strive to become the kind of surgeon others want to operate and collaborate with because your cases unfold smoothly, and on those occasions when a case hits a roadblock, you remain calm, cool, and in control.

No, I am not advising you to keep your emotions and feelings pent up all the time under trying circumstances. I admit, when things take a turn for the worse in the OR, I drop some F-bombs to get it out of my system, but I shift quickly back to the task at hand. I take care to direct all the F-bombs at me, and not anyone else in the room. In fact, I cannot recall at time when I ever cursed anyone else out in the operating room.

Yes, you will deal with trying cases.

You will have moments when you think to yourself, "Oh my gosh, what have I gotten myself into?" You are only human. But if you stay focused and calm, you will give yourself the best chance at success.

CHAPTER 3 PRESCRIPTIONS FOR A HEALTHY PRACTICE

❖ Have another surgeon join you on challenging cases.

❖ Always portray a sense of confidence and control.

❖ Remain calm all the time.

❖ Schedule cases for more time than you anticipate.

QUESTIONS TO CONSIDER...REMEMBER, STAYING IN CONTROL OF YOUR EMOTIONS IS VITAL

1. Do I regularly time my surgeries so I know how long it takes me to do my bread and butter cases?

_____

_____

_____

_____

_____

_____

_____

2. Am I under or over the times I book my cases for?

_____

_____

_____

_____

_____

_____

_____

3. When a case becomes stressful, how do I react? Do I stay calm and cool or spazz out on a regular basis?

_____

_____

_____

_____

_____

_____

_____

4. Do I consistently evaluate how I handle tough cases?

_____

_____

_____

_____

_____

_____

_____

5. What am I doing to get better at handling stress in the OR? When an unforeseen challenge arises again, how will I react?

_____

_____

_____

_____

_____

_____

_____

Chapter 4

Maintain a Smooth-Running Office

Most young surgeons coming out into practice want to become exceptional surgeons. Well, to become an exceptional surgeon you must operate on a significant number of patients. To operate on a significant number of patients, you must see a significant number of patients in clinic. To achieve this goal, you must implement systems that allow you to increase your patient load while still providing excellent care. Ten percent of the patients we see in my clinic choose to have an operation. If my goal is to perform 500 surgeries per year, I must book 10 cases per week. That means I must see roughly 100 patients a week in the office.

It always surprises me that surgeons do not possess a better grasp of these numbers. If you want to assume the persona of a Dr. Hustle, the first thing you must do is determine the number of cases you want to take on in a year. Maybe it is 100 or 1,000. It is not the actual number of cases that matters because that is an individual choice. What matters is for you to gain clarity on your annual goal. Once you have a number in mind, work backwards to figure out what actions you must take in the clinic to achieve it. If you want to build a thriving surgical practice, developing and maintaining office efficiency is a requirement. I liken efficiency in the office to installing the fiberoptic cables into your practice *before* you need the one gig of bandwidth. Prepare for future traffic jams by building the infrastructure first.

Too many young surgeons wait until they get a little busy. The next thing they know, they are running more than an hour behind before they focus on improving clinic efficiency. Playing catch-up plain sucks – for you, your MA, and most importantly, your patients. People *hate* seeing a doctor that runs behind all the time and doctors hate the feeling of being behind. To avoid this outcome, brainstorm ways to handle the volume of patients you desire in an efficient manner that supports and maintains your quality of care.

Here is a simple principle I adhere to: spend the maximum amount of time in the examining room with patients and a minimal amount of time outside the room not talking to patients. If you do this in a consistent manner, you will improve your efficiency and maintain high-quality care. You must be in the examining room talking, interacting, examining, and thinking about patients – not in the middle of the workstation dealing with your EMR or any other issues in clinic that can be delegated. Your most valuable time is spent with your patients – everything else can be delegated. Keep the necessity of staying in the rooms with your patients top-of-mind. When I was a fellow, one of my mentors drilled this into my head. He was among the most efficient surgeons I ever worked with and his happy patients expressed the utmost satisfaction with him.

Yes, we face a common conundrum: our patients want us to take our time with them and not feel rushed, yet on the other hand, our practices have built-in cost constraints. Many of us in private practice are not just orthopedic surgeons but entrepreneurs running a business and we must consider our fixed overhead costs. To make your payroll and pay the lease or mortgage on your building, there is a minimum number of patients you must see to generate the required surgical volume. People often criticize surgeons for seeing too many patients: *How can they spend enough time with them? Do they really care about their patients or is it all about the money?* Everyone has their comfort zone with respect to the speed with which they move through clinic. It is a huge range.

For example, I recall in vivid detail when I was a medical student working with a neurologist at a university hospital who spent four solid hours talking to one single patient in the morning. She even booked the appointment for four hours! I could not believe it. Most of us would agree that is on the far end of the spectrum where we do not want to be. On the flip side, when I was a fellow, I worked with a surgeon who regularly saw 100 patients in a day, twice a week, with one fellow and one nurse. We would get done between 3:00 and 3:30 in the afternoon.

Some doctors or surgeons may scoff at this kind of volume, believing a surgeon who crams that many patients into their daily schedule does them a disservice. How can you possibly maintain a high standard of care when you see all those patients in one day? Well, we are all wired differently, and our minds think differently. If that surgeon has an office full of 100 patients, it is likely many of them are satisfied with his results. Particularly if you are in private practice, if you do not do good work and provide a great patient experience, you will not have a busy office.

Of course, there is a limit to what each one of us can do in terms of our ability to provide safe, high-quality care. We must have ample time to make proper decisions. However, as you gain experience your mind moves at a much faster pace; therefore, it takes less time to determine what you must do. Your first six months- to- one year in practice are not like you second, third, fifth, or tenth year. We all continue to evolve and things that required a significant amount of thought in the beginning do not demand as much time and thought in the end. You will encounter multiple situations in your practice but as you continue to grow as a surgeon, the things that you wracked your brain over in the early years will become second-nature. When you confront these scenarios, you will know in an instant what to do.

Yes, patients will walk through your doors with a pathology you have never seen before, but that is what makes our field exciting. As you gain experience, see more patients, and build your volume, these situations will become fewer and farther between. Once you feel comfortable enough and have established certain algorithms for treatment, you can increase your efficiency by delegating specific tasks.

In my clinic, for example, I have little interaction with my staff during hours. I go into examining rooms, where I spend 90 percent of my time interacting with patients. I use iScribe, a virtual scribe service, to dictate my notes, which I typically do while the patient is in the room, unless I fall a bit behind. My virtual scribe transcribes the dictation. They put in all the ICP 10 and CPT codes. I scribble down in shorthand on a piece of paper for my MA anything I need. Then, I move to the next room while my MA works on whatever I described in the note.

When ordering tasks (PT, prescriptions, tests, surgery), I've found that writing directives on a piece of paper and putting it on the door – versus trying to find someone to tell them verbally – is a much more efficient process. Another effective practice we have implemented is numbering each one of the doors in the clinic, so I know which rooms to go in next. I am not thinking about what the order is, and I can minimize wait times by going to the patient who is the first in line. My nurse places little clips on the door labeled 1, 2, 3, 4. As soon as I come out of the room, I look for number one.

A NOTE ON VIRTUAL SCRIBES

Virtual scribes have proven to be one of the biggest efficiency hacks in my office. My virtual scribed literally shaved an hour-and-a-half off my EMR usage each day, which not only gets me home earlier but allows me to see more patients. At the same time, I feel less rushed in clinic and provide better quality care because I spend less time interacting with the computer and more time interacting with people.

The scribe service is simple. As with traditional methods, I dictate into a phone; however, the difference with a virtual scribe is that they automatically input the CPT codes, ICD-10, and follow-ups, so you do not have to touch the computer. The note is ready within 20 minutes and then you sign in. For the first several years of my practice, I used Dragon, which worked okay. But there were many errors in the Dragon dictation that forced me to go back and edit, which was frustrating because it slowed me down too much in clinic.

You can choose to hire an in-person scribe. I opted for a virtual scribe because there is a high turnover rate with human scribes, plus you must deal with the headaches that go along with hiring another employee. In the current digital age, we can outsource many things; entrepreneurs employ virtual assistants all over the world. Thus, a virtual scrive is just another virtual assistant for you and your office. They are physically in the EMR, inputting the codes and the dictation. The best part about the service is that it features a much friendlier user interface and can interface with any EMR in existence. I highly recommend that you research one of these services.

Automate as many tasks as you can. For your common clinic visit or two-week post-op, create one-word templates or pre-set templates where you can either finish the entire note with the click of a button or the utterance of one word. This will increase your speed significantly. I follow the same process for my common surgeries. When I book someone for a shoulder replacement, for example, I simply say, "shoulder arthroplasty surgery," and the scribe knows to input in the full paragraph explaining all the risks, benefits, etc.

ONE TEAM ALIGNED WITH A SHARED VISION

Before you can train your MA to delegate all appropriate tasks, you must have an honest conversation with them about your vision and objectives. When I first started my practice, I informed my MA of my goals from a patient volume standpoint. At first, she looked at me as if to say, "Are you serious?"

"I understand that is a huge number of patients and volume," I replied, "but that is where I want to go. If that is not where you want to go, maybe we should part ways now."

Despite her initial reaction, she fully accepted and understood my expectations for our office. As a result of our frank discussion and her complete alignment with my vision, we developed an amazing working relationship and achieved our shared goals. To manifest your vision for your practice, you must first conceive of it in detail in your mind, then share your vision with your staff to ensure that they are in total alignment and understand their role in contributing to the success of the practice.

From there, you must develop the habit of delegating a significant amount of authority to your MAs and PAs. The more trust you can place in your staff by delegating tasks, the more your practice will thrive. Delegating tasks accomplishes two main objectives: it frees you up to do the things that *only* you can do, and it instills a sense of purpose and autonomy within your employees because they understand how important they are to the success of the practice. In general, people are much happier in the workplace when they are empowered to make decisions and believe that their role makes a crucial contribution to your mission. Create a great system, hire good people to work in it, and do your best to get out of their way.

As your practice grows, mistakes will be made, requiring you to train your MA to perform certain tasks. However, most of the time they will impress you with their abilities. If not, you must consider hiring a new MA. As the old saying goes, *"Hire slow, fire fast."* Several of my partners have dealt with MAs who simply could not keep up with the amount of volume in their practice. It became a constant battle, and, in the end, they had to part ways. It is a difficult decision to fire any member of your staff because you develop a close relationship with them over the years.

You can avoid this unpleasant outcome by following my advice above: develop a clear, detailed vision for your practice that includes the number of patients you want to see and the number of surgeries you want to perform. You may start with an MA who worked with another surgeon for years whose practice saw only 25 to 30 patients a day. If your goal is see 50 patients a day, the MA may respond by telling you that is crazy and finding another job. Or they may respond with enthusiasm because they were bored in their previous job and embrace the idea working for a busy practice. Until you initiate an honest conversation with them about the goals you have set for your practice, you cannot know for sure if they are a good fit.

Remember, there are all sorts of medical practices out there and all kinds of orthopedic surgeons. If the MA (or any member of your staff) does not align with your vision, you do them a disservice by hiring and/or keeping them employed. It only hurts you and them. Once you determine it is mutually beneficial to let them go, rip off the Band-Aid. It will be painful, but the faster you do it, the better.

PRE-OP APPOINTMENTS, SECOND OPINIONS, AND OTHER WAYS TO CREATE EFFICIENCY

Another beneficial policy my practice has implemented is to schedule pre-op appointments for our patients. It has resulted in greater efficiency, especially for larger operations such as rotator cuff repairs, arthroplasties, and complex procedures. These pre-op appointments assist us in getting our patients their prescriptions, slings, and pre-op antibacterial washes, and answering their questions about surgery. When they show up in the operating room, they have no questions because they already reviewed the information multiple times and written it down. We can enter the OR with confidence that the patient is fully educated and informed about what is going to transpire. It is much easier to do that in the office in a calm environment than in the preoperative area when everybody is nervous. In addition, a pre-operative appointment offers an excellent opportunity to introduce patients to your PA if your PA will be making the rounds.

If you are seeing a patient who is seeking a second opinion, or has had another operation, train your staff to obtain all the images and documents, and load them into your PACS system (most of us have an electronic radiology system these days). Before you meet the patient in your office, everything must be scanned and loaded into your PACS so you can access it ahead of time. We make it a habit not to rely on other offices. Tell your patients to bring their own imaging to the appointment because often other offices will drop the ball.

A final note on clinic efficiency: you must measure what you do. In my practice, we review patient wait times, the volume of patients we see, and the number of negative comments we receive. We use a service with our online marketing agency that texts our patients for feedback after every visit, which enables us to ascertain what we must improve with much more clarity. The instant we get negative feedback, I receive an email. We record our results within our practice and discuss them during our partner meetings to determine how we stack up against them. This provides us objective criteria that helps us to measure our results.

CHAPTER 4 PRESCRIPTIONS FOR A HEALTHY PRACTICE

❖ Always take time to talk to patients.

❖ Virtual and personal scribes are essential.

❖ Automate procedures as much as you can.

❖ The more you delegate, the more efficient you become.

QUESTIONS TO CONSIDER...REMEMBER, THE CLEARER YOUR VISION, THE GREATER YOUR ABILITY TO IDENTIFY AND RETAIN STAFF THAT ALIGN WITH IT

1. What specific number of patients do I want to see in my clinic? Why? Have I shared my expectations with my entire staff?

_____

_____

_____

_____

_____

_____

2. Do I have the "bandwidth" to see the number of patients I must see to achieve my desired volume of surgery? If not, what can I do to go from dial up speeds to fiberoptic speeds?

_____

_____

_____

_____

_____

_____

3. Have I hired a PA? If I have the volume to justify it, what is stopping me?

_____

_____

_____

_____

_____

_____

4. If I already have a PA, how can I utilize them more efficiently in my clinic? Am I delegating to them or micro-managing them?

_____

_____

_____

_____

_____

_____

5. Do I sit down with my team on a regular basis to discuss ways to improve efficiency and the overall patient experience?

_____

_____

_____

_____

_____

_____

6. How I measure your results? Do I track my patient volumes, wait times, and actively seek feedback from my patients?

_____

_____

_____

_____

_____

_____

Chapter 5

Hire a Physician Assistant and OR Assistants

Most of us completed different fellowships and residencies, where we interacted with PAs on a regular basis that worked in busy and mature surgical practices and sub-specialized practices. Some surgical practices did not employ PAs. The choice to hire a PA is up to you; however, after reading this chapter, if you have not already hired a PA, you most likely will.

Aside from improving the overall quality of your practice, the countless benefits of employing a PA include the ability to:

➤ Scale your practice

➤ Delegate tasks

➤ Increase your volume

➤ Enhance your all-around efficiency as a surgeon

In most businesses, it is a general rule that as the owner/entrepreneur (in this case, YOU, the surgeon) become busier, you must learn how to delegate certain tasks to others, while you focus on the job that only you can do – perform complex surgeries and make vital medical decisions on behalf of your patients. When you are in the office, your valuable time must be spent managing the pathology of your patients and determining who to operate on and not to operate on. These are just a few examples of the numerous functions that only you can fulfill.

However, there is a long list of tasks that your support staff can take on, and the better you delegate them, the more efficient your practice becomes. It is arduous to develop a thriving practice without help; therefore, you must learn how to hire, train, and assemble good people around you that will allow you to practice medicine in the most effective way possible.

However, if you are just coming out of practice, it is not in your best interest to hire a PA right away. First, you are not that busy and do not yet have the volume to justify it. More than likely, you and your PA will end up sitting around and staring at each other while you twiddle your thumbs for the first year or two. Second, you have boards to deal with. During boards, you must be hypervigilant about your notes and coding. You must place your hands on all those patients and put in the dictations and notes. Can you imagine meeting the ABOS and trying to explain a bunch of notes written by your PA? Not a good idea. Finally, it is impossible to teach a PA about your practice and your preferences for accomplishing certain things, if you have not defined that for yourself. For most surgeons, it takes a year or two in practice to figure it out.

Now, as it pertains to the OR, it benefits you to have some sort of help when you are in the early stages of your practice. Depending on the structure of your practice, your group or hospital may have already hired PAs that are readily available for you in the OR. If that is the case, awesome. If not, a more streamlined approach would be to get a certified first assistant that covers your cases. If I could go back in time, I would do things differently. For the first several years of my practice, I employed an excellent first assist until I felt like I had reached a point where I could justify a PA salary. Although the PA I hired did a wonderful job, they collected a tremendous amount of money from my cases that I did not collect. As with anyone else who piggybacks on something you do in the clinic, that revenue flows directly from cases you generate. Most surgeons bill for their PAs and keep any excess revenue for themselves.

That is how all businesses work, and a surgical practice is no different. At the outset of your practice, if you do not have access to PAs or first assists through your group, you must hire one on your own. Set up an LLC where you bill and code for the first assist. The first assist gets paid either by case or as a percentage of collection, and you keep the rest. This system generates a significant amount of monthly income, which means everybody wins: the first assist gets work, and you get a portion of the excess revenue. In addition, if you hire a first assist who has experience, you do not have to worry about training them.

It becomes even more efficient when first assists work with multiple other surgeons. If your first assist works with two- to- three surgeons, you pay them a percentage of collections by case or an agreed-upon amount per case. Either way, you only pay one person what they are worth, and establish a fixed amount of overhead. First assists typically earn between $60,000 to $100,000 a year. Anything generated over this amount is profit, and you can generate a significant amount of revenue by hiring a first assist. That said, the downside is that they can only help you in the operating room and, like most surgeons, you probably need help in the clinic, too.

Once you reach the point where you believe a PA could help from a clinical perspective, convert to hiring a PA. Sure, it is fantastic to have help in the operating room; however, you will not generate more surgeries unless you can handle more volume in the office. That is where a PA can make a tremendous impact on increasing your volume by seeing patients in your office while you are not there or are tending to other cases.

How Do You Determine When It Is Time to Hire a PA in the Office?

This can be a complex question and one many surgeons grapple with. If you polled 100 orthopedic surgeons on when they got their PA, if they got their PA too soon, or if they waited too long to get a PA, 99 percent of them would say they waited too long. Most of us are worried about the cost and whether we can justify the use of a PA; hence, we probably wait too long to get one. However, you should hire a PA *sooner* than you think. When you analyze the numbers, the amount of money a PA can collect from surgery, and how much they can help you crank up your office volume *and* maintain a high standard of patient care, it only makes sense pay for a PA.

Most PAs in our practice generate revenue for us, which is incredible: you have an employee who helps you increase your volume, see more patients, perform surgery in less time, and spend more time with your family – and you make money from it! It almost seems too good to be true, and as with most things in life, you must accept, understand, and watch for certain trade-offs. For example, PAs only get reimbursed for reimbursable cases in the operating room. Simply put, if you replace a joint, fix a fracture, or repair something, that is a reimbursable surgery. All other surgeries typically do not get reimbursed. These include a simple knee scope meniscectomy, carpal tunnels, and many hand/wrist and foot/ankle cases, along with other sub-specialties of orthopedics. I am not suggesting you should not use a PA for these types of cases, just offering a word of caution that your volume must be higher than the other specialties, and that you must employ your PA more in the office than in the OR to enable them to generate the revenue necessary to cover their salary.

Keep in mind, some of the more trauma-heavy cases such as hip; knee; spine; foot and ankle; and other sports cases involving repairs get reimbursed, but generally not as much as some of the other subspecialties. Before you hire a PA take this into consideration. In addition, you must ask yourself: "How much am I willing to pay for this PA, and how much are they going to help me?"

Set that number and go backwards. Once you decide to hire a PA, the question becomes a matter of experience. Should you hire a seasoned PA or one fresh out of school? A seasoned PA comes with many advantages:

they have already been vetted, they know how to work, and they will not demand as much of your time for training. On the flip side, you may have to un-train some of the things they learned from other doctors to operate in a way that best suits your practice. Furthermore, their experience commands a higher salary, whereas a PA right out of school will start off at a much lower salary. Whether experienced or new, the market in your area will also influence their salary.

With a PA who is just embarking upon their career, you will invest time teaching them. However, your investment will pay off because your PA will be trained in your ways from the get-go, and you'll still pay them less than an experienced PA. In my case, my PA was regularly seeing patients on her own, rounding, and closing all incisions in the operating room with excellence within six months, and I know she is only going to get better.

Every PA is unique. You must interview them. You must vet them. Hiring someone directly out of school is a bit risky because you have no precedent as to how they work; therefore, you must be careful during the interview process. I feel fortunate to have an excellent PA who has been an awesome fit for my practice. Because she had also done a rotation with one of my partners, he got to see her work first-hand. He was so impressed, he insisted we hire her as a group. At the time, I was not sure I was ready for a PA, but the decision to hire her has been one of the best I have made in my practice thus far.

THE PA: ROCKET FUEL FOR YOUR CLINIC'S EFFICIENCY

Once again, a PA can be an asset to an efficient practice *if* you learn how to delegate. As with the MA, the more you delegate and trust, the more efficient you will be. However, you cannot just turn your PA loose; you must be willing to train them. There is a huge difference between *delegating*, giving a task to someone to perform on your behalf; and *abdicating*, handing off a task and running away. To reiterate, the goal is to delegate as much as you can so you can spend more time making complex decisions, planning operations, and trouble-shooting any problems that arise. You want to spend most of your time engaged in the activities that only you can do.

One of my favorite sayings is, "Let bad little things happen so great big things can happen," a philosophy that applies to hiring a PA in your practice. The bad little things are the discomfort of giving up control and dealing with some patients' complaints about not getting to see the doctor (typical with older patients). The great big things are a massive efficiency boost for your practice. You can see more patients in less time and provide a better patient experience overall. Patients can be worked into your clinic faster because your PA handles the straightforward cases that can be delegated (post ops, follow ups, simple new patients), which frees you up to see the more complex patients that require operations. You will spend *more* time with patients whose issues demand your expertise and experience.

As I mentioned, I can guarantee that some of your patients will complain about seeing a PA and not the doctor. In my practice, we address the problem by being forthcoming about the kind of patients my PA takes care of. If the patient responds that they would still rather see the doctor, we assure them that is perfectly fine; however, there will be fewer available time slots and possibly longer wait times. Then we let them decide. This policy helps the patient understand why you hired a PA in the first place, and that there is a trade-off. By letting the patient decide, we have cut down on the complaints considerably. Think of your PA as an extension of yourself: when you put it in the framework, bringing on a PA not only allows the practice to see more patients, but to take better care of them. When trained and utilized appropriately, PAs increase quantity and quality.

One valid concern for young surgeons is the cost of a PA. Various groups handle it in different ways, but for the most part PAs generate more than enough in revenue to compensate for their salary and benefits – and even if they didn't, the efficiencies they create in your practice more than make up for any small losses. In our practice, PA salaries range from $90,000 to $180,000, and most of them more than compensate for that in revenue.

CHAPTER 5 PRESCRIPTIONS FOR A HEALTHY PRACTICE

❖ As you get busier, you must learn how to delegate certain tasks.

❖ Be shrewd about the way you allow first assists to help you.

❖ Get a PA sooner than you think.

❖ Learn to let go so others can help you.

❖ Once you hire a PA, give them as much autonomy as possible to free you up to do the things only you can do.

QUESTIONS TO CONSIDER...REMEMBER, HIRING THE RIGHT PA WILL PROPEL YOU TO GREATER SUCCESS

1. If I do not have a PA yet, what volume do I need to justify it? (it is lower than most surgeons think)

_____

_____

_____

_____

_____

_____

2. If I have the volume to justify and cover a PA's salary, why haven't I hired one yet?

_____

_____

_____

_____

_____

_____

3. If I have a PA do I have a system in place to allow patients to choose whether they will see the PA or the doctor to avoid complaints?

_____

_____

_____

_____

_____

_____

4. If I have a PA am I micromanaging them, or empowering them to make decisions?

_____

_____

_____

_____

_____

_____

5. If I am in the first two years of practice do I a first assist helping me with cases regularly? If so have I set up an LLC so that the payment for the cases come to *me* first, then they get a percentage or set payment per case?

_____

_____

_____

_____

_____

_____

Chapter 6

Keep the Sword Sharp

It is imperative that you continue to evolve as a surgeon. It enables you to create niches in the market and set yourself apart from others. Two of the most important things you can and should do is attend conferences and read journals within your sub-specialty. Once you establish your practice, it is up to you to focus on your professional development and grow with the times. Go to as many conferences as you can. The highest value you will receive from your attendance is the opportunity to meet, network, and nurture relationships with other surgeons. These relationships will enable you to bounce ideas, solicit their advice for difficult cases, and discover what your peers are doing. Every time I go to a conference, I come home with five different things I want to change in my practice.

Naturally, my office and the OR roll their eyes every time I come back with a desire to switch things up a bit. In some ways, it is a double-edged sword because the more you change, the more difficult it can be to maintain efficiency, but on the other hand, you cannot keep doing the same things over and over. Additionally, the goal of the new processes is to improve efficiency, so once we get through the initial learning curve operations will be smoother. Surgeons that maintain the status quo in their practice do not remain busy. As the trendy quote goes, you must learn how to "become comfortable being a little bit uncomfortable". You must make subtle changes and tweaks to your practice and stay hungry and sharp. Attending conferences and reading two- to-three journals to within your sub-specialty monthly will give you an edge and distinguish you from 90 percent of surgeons in terms of up-to-date knowledge.

Utilize Cadaver Labs

Cadaver labs offer an excellent opportunity to hone your skills and prepare for surgery, yet they tend to be underused by orthopedic surgeons. If you are going to employ a new technique, leverage the reps around you, most of whom are happy to buy you a cadaver, and bring it to your OR for a typical cost of about $500. I often use cadavers to practice the surgery I plan to perform the next day or week in my operating room. Most hospitals allow it, and cadavers are no less sterile than a live human being – actually, a cadaver is more sterile because it has been embalmed and most likely has less bacteria than a live person. I instruct my staff to wash a few of the trays we used for surgery and keep them around. Then I ask the reps bring in the cadavers and get to work. You can also leverage cadavers for surgeries that do not require implants.

It is an excellent way to prepare for surgeries because you are in your environment, with the reps and staff that will be there for the actual case. When you practice on a cadaver, you will always encounter an issue that you did not envision going wrong in surgery. You are in your OR performing the surgery, just like you will be with the live patient, so everything looks and feels the same, including your tools and equipment. The sight and smell of the room is the same. As you can attest from your prior work on cadavers as a fellow and resident, it is harder than working on a person. However, operating on a cadaver is a great way to practice performing new surgeries and employing novel techniques.

Given these advantages, it surprises me that other orthopedic surgeons do not make it a habit to operate on cadavers. Instead, they "wing it" on a patient. We surgeons tend to feel like we can get that done (which is true), but why not work out many of the kinks on a cadaver first? You can operate much more smoothly on your patient the next day, as I can attest from my own experience.

Furthermore, when I have difficult operations scheduled that I do not perform on a regular basis that do not require implants, I'll tell the reps to bring me a cadaver. I leverage my relationships with my reps with the knowledge that I use many of their implants. They make a significant amount of money off me; therefore, they will bring me a cadaver, even if though they do not make any money from it if they want to keep my business. In the long run, it is a huge win for the reps. However, the case itself will pay for the cost of the cadaver most of the time. Do not feel guilty about asking your rep to buy you a cadaver: they are dying to get the one-on-one time with you to sell you on their products. Take advantage of it and learn!

Elbow arthroscopy is a technically challenging operation that does not come around frequently, especially in the early stages of your practice. Since I was well-trained in elbow arthroscopy as a fellow, I had the opportunity to work on these cases when I first started out in practice. However, for every single elbow scope I did in my first two years, I asked the reps bring in an elbow the night before I scoped the elbow on the person, and practiced for an hour and a half the night before in my operating room, with my equipment, with the reps. We set up everything, including all the equipment. Most times, my assistant stayed with me, which made the operations unfold much more smoothly. As the adage goes, "repetition is the mother of skill." With every procedure we completed, the better we got.

SPECIALIZE, SPECIALIZE, SPECIALIZE

The more you specialize in an area and the more you repeat the same operations, the better you get. You understand pathology better. You become more efficient at the simple things, but you can also recognize when something fits outside the box. You get to see more of the weird pathology more frequently, so you can look back on it and say to yourself, "If I have seen 5,000 shoulders versus 100 shoulders, I'm going to see the unusual stuff more often. I'm going to know how to handle these things."

Deciding what to take on and what not to take on in your practice presents a bit of a conundrum. That is a personal decision you must make. You should take on challenging cases early on in your practice, so long as you feel confident you can get the job done. If you can accept demanding cases and accomplish excellent results early on, it will help you in tremendous ways. Other surgeons will regard you as a problem solver. They will look at you as a garbage can because you embrace the things that they do not like to do. Their trash is your treasure. Whether it is a case in their office they do not like or a complication they do not want to resolve, you want to be the surgeon that solves their problem.

For instance, in my practice, I came into a group of seven sports doctors who all did shoulder surgery, but, fortunately for me, none of them wanted to do replacements, complex revisions of instability, revisions of rotator cuff repairs, bad fractures, revision shoulder arthroplasty, etc. I took on all these things for the group from an early period. Yes, it was difficult to handle that influx of complex cases, but it made me a much better surgeon, and revved up my skill process quickly. You must be willing to take on such cases, but you must first ask yourself, "Can I do a good job?"

If you genuinely feel like you cannot do it, refer it out. Once you feel confident in your ability to handle complex cases with precision and excellence, the more you take on, the faster your practice will grow. The key lies in your competency – which hinges upon regular attendance at conferences, conversations with different surgeons, and the development a network of peers with whom you can bounce ideas and discuss individual cases. Oftentimes, tough cases involve good decision-making and preparation on the front end more than a high level of technical skill.

If you take my advice, you will set yourself apart from many orthopedic surgeons in the community. It is easy to become complacent within our profession because you make so much money doing simple operations. That said, there is a cost. If you do that for 15- to- 20 years, all the sudden you will become irrelevant. There will be more competition in the market for the easy cases. You do not make more money from doing revision cases and complex cases than you do simple cases in the short term. In fact, you make way less money when you consider the time, effort, and energy that it takes to handle complicated cases, compared to the straightforward ones.

In my case, a 1-cm rotator cuff tears pay the same as massive, retracted tears where I must do a patch or a graft or some other type of operation to fix them. However, by being the "expert" or "problem solver" for the community, I have created a reputation that enables me to receive all the complex cases and accept patients with demanding problems. These patients then broadcast my name to the community as an orthopedic surgeon who solved their issue when no one else could.

When you succeed with a patient whose previous surgeon and surgery failed, it gives you an invaluable marketing tool to build and expand your practice. Believe it or not, the most efficient referral source you can ever get is another orthopedic surgeon. I repeat: *the most efficient referral source you can get is another orthopedic surgeon.* When your orthopedic peer refers a patient to you, 99.9 percent of the time, it is a surgical patient.

As we have discussed previously, five- to- 10 percent of the patients you see will result in surgery. That is the rule-of-thumb. Primary doctors, therapists, chiropractors, and other non-orthopedic referral sources cannot ascertain when a patient's issue requires surgery, whereas an orthopedic surgeon most likely can. When an orthopedic surgeon sends you a patient, chances are it is because that patient needs an operation the orthopedic surgeon does not want to perform. If you operate successfully on their patient, they see you as a problem solver. When the next patient comes along with a similar issue, that orthopedic surgeon will think, "I want this person out of my office. I am going to send them back to that doctor." Multiple orthopedic surgeons around the community that have done that for me.

Every time I see their name, I know it is a surgical patient. An orthopedic surgeon is the most difficult referral source to obtain, but once you reach that level, it will increase your cases with maximum efficiency. However, you must have the capacity to deal well with demanding, complicated problems. It is easy to convince a PCP that they should send patients to you, the new young guy in town, but it is much more difficult to convince another orthopedic surgeon to send you operative cases because they are much stricter in their assessment of your abilities.

Choose your niche area, then become the surgeon that handles the disaster cases for that specific area or type of operation. If you can develop that reputation, you're going to obtain those referral sources; those patients are going to tell their friends about you; and they're going to send the business you want. At that point, you will get the easy chip shot total knee and total hip. You will get the ACL tear in the seventeen-year-old girl if you can handle the HTO with a cartilage restoration in her forty-one-year-old mother.

➢ You are known as the complex hip and knee arthroplasty surgeon.

➢ You are known as the shoulder surgeon.

➢ You are known as the elbow surgeon.

➢ You are known as the surgeon around town that handles the complex problems nobody else wants to deal with.

These patients are difficult to deal with, and their surgeries present extreme demands and stress, but someone must do them. If you can make yourself that person, it will quickly grow your practice. Why doesn't everybody do this? It is hard. It is painful. It is stressful. It hurts sometimes when these patients have complications (which they will no matter how good you are).

I always tell one of my partners, "You can either be a bit stressed out in your clinic by pushing yourself to see more patients, and a bit stressed out in the OR by successfully performing complex surgeries nobody else wants to do, or you can be stressed out at the end of the month when you look at the number of cases you did and how much you collected."

Many of my partners trade being stressed out in the clinic from high patient volume or in the OR due to taxing operations for short-term peace-of-mind. The trade-off comes at the end of the month when we review our collections. Then, they feel stressed. The point is you can choose the reason for your stress. I prefer to be a bit stressed out about seeing more patients in the office and doing high-level complex surgery on several patients than being unhappy with my take-home pay. The more exhausted I am when I come home from clinic and the OR, the bigger the check at the end of the month.

As you move forward in your career, you will be surprised that the things that created stress for you in your first year versus your fifth year are not even close. Push the limits of what you can do and grind out little things on a continual basis. A massive, retracted rotator cuff tear for me in my first year of practice took me two hours – something I can now do in under an hour. I forced myself to take on complex tears and fix them, and now I can handle a small tear with my eyes closed. If you do the complex stuff consistently, the straightforward cases become so easy, you feel like you could do them in your sleep. You do not even have to think anymore.

Of course, you must focus on performing your best surgery, no matter the type of case. However, when you push yourself to do the hard stuff, the easy stuff becomes second nature to you. It is fun. The same is true for the complicated stuff. Revision shoulder arthroplasty was the most difficult thing I did, but now that I've gotten 20 or 30 under my belt, I look forward to those cases because I know how to fix the problems that can come along with them.

As I discussed before in the OR chapter, once you learn to resolve a problematic situation such as an intraoperative fracture or a vessel that bleeds more than you would like, you can tuck the solution away in your hard drive for future operations. You can relax because you have been there before, and you know how to deal with it. In the beginning, as you move through the pain of the learning curve, the first few will suck. You will endure some sleepless nights. The more sleepless nights you have (especially early on), the greater you will develop an ability to handle the unexpected with precision and care. Most surgeons do not want to perform challenging surgeries, but someone has help these patients resolve their issues. If you are the guy or girl who can do that, you will set yourself apart from your peers. It requires a tremendous amount of effort, diligence, self-knowledge, and a willingness to learn how to resolve complex problems, but once you do, you will be way ahead of the game.

Keep your sword sharp. Continue to work on your surgical skills and refine your technique. Take notes on all the surgeries you have done when you come home at night. Examine any problems you experience, evolve, and change your approach to become better and more efficient. When I first started doing shoulder arthroplasty, my cases took me over an hour-and-a-half to go skin-to-skin. Now, an average shoulder arthroplasty takes me roughly 40 to 45 minutes. Why? I have performed a huge amount of them – including rather difficult ones – and I have an excellent team helping me.

STRIVE TO BE AN EFFICIENT SURGEON

In our practice, we consistently analyze cases and brainstorm ways to be more efficient in our operations. We remove unnecessary parts of every procedure, yet we never rush. If you rush, it goes slower; therefore, you cannot attempt to be a "fast" surgeon. One of the best quotes I ever heard was from a guy named Jim Strickland, a world-renown hand surgeon, who told me that the fellows always came to him with a desire to become a fast surgeon. He said, "You don't become a fast surgeon by *trying* to be a fast surgeon. You became a fast surgeon by being an efficient surgeon, and efficient surgery is the systematic elimination of unnecessary parts of the procedure."

An efficient surgeon understands how to eliminate unneeded aspects of a procedure. If you witness a surgery and exclaim, "Oh my God, I can't believe how fast that went," you have seen an excellent surgeon at work. It should almost appear as if they are in slow motion – there is little wasted movement, and everything goes where it is supposed to go. To reach peak surgical efficiency, you must evaluate every operation you perform and ask, "What parts of the procedure take us a long time? How can we smooth it out? What unnecessary steps can we eliminate to achieve the same result?"

You do not become a fast surgeon by being sloppy or skipping *necessary* steps. Efficient, smooth surgeons always ask themselves, "How can I do this smoother and quicker?" A non-surgeon might hear a surgeon brag, "I did a shoulder replacement in 30 minutes," and think, "Oh my gosh, that surgeon rushes through his operations. That is dangerous." If someone said this to me, I would reply, "Would it make you feel better if I said it took me four hours?"

Rest assured; I will never compromise the results of my surgery for 10,000 reasons. However, I see a problem with a surgeon that takes 45 minutes to do a carpal tunnel when it takes someone else five minutes and they both arrive at the same result; or a surgeon that takes two hours to do a total knee when other surgeons can do it in 30- to- 45 minutes. The same principle applies to every operation.

Surgical literature reveals that the longer the patient is open on the operating table, the greater their chances of having a problem such as an infection or another complication. You could argue that the length of time it takes you to perform an operation depends upon its complexity and multiple other factors, which is true. However, even when accounting for these scenarios, the longer an operation takes to complete, the greater the number of complications it will present.

When I was in residency, one of my mentors always told us that operating rooms are not sterile. Although they are clean, there is bacteria in the air. If you can do an operation in one-third the time and achieve the same result, you should strive to do that every time. According to the trends, our field is moving in that direction. With an aging population, we can bet on having to resolve more problems for more people via surgery. In 10 years, for example, the number of arthroplasties we perform right now is going to double. And more than likely we will get paid less to do them, which means you must develop smoother processes that result in efficient operations. A huge component of achieving that goal is to evaluate yourself as a surgeon, be diligent about your performance, and grade yourself with brutal honesty. Review your tourniquet times, your X-rays, and your results. Make it a habit to measure, analyze, and improve.

An outcomes database offers an objective method of measuring your outcomes. There are multiple systems available, but I utilize SOS from Arthrex. Although these systems require little time from you, they benefit you for many reasons – first and foremost because you cannot improve upon something without an objective measurement tool. If you do not track your outcomes, how can you know if you are getting better or not? Second, many of the payers will require this in the future; it is better to get started now than be forced to do it later. Finally, tracking your outcomes provides an effective marketing tool. I publish outcomes for my common operations on my website and discuss them with my patients. It is great to be able to look someone in the eye and tell them exactly what your outcomes are for a particular procedure and not just quote something from the literature (different surgeon, different patients). This entire process takes me no more than two minutes per patient. I plug the info in when I am sitting at the computer doing my post-op orders. The patients get an email before and after surgery to track their progress. Best of all, you can review a change you made in surgery to determine if it affected your outcomes, enabling you to be much more objective about the changes you implement.

If you continually sharpen your sword, your patients will do better, and you will set yourself apart from your peers. Learning does not stop when you become a fellow – on the contrary, it begins. You must treat your practice like a 30-year fellowship, do new things, and evolve.

CHAPTER 6 PRESCRIPTIONS FOR A HEALTHY PRACTICE

- ❖ Learn how to become comfortable being a bit uncomfortable.

- ❖ Use cadavers to prepare for complicated surgeries.

- ❖ Become a specialist as much as possible.

- ❖ Learn to deal with complex problems.

- ❖ Keep your sword sharp with constant learning and improving.

- ❖ Choose to be an efficient surgeon, not a fast one. Avoid sloppiness and skipping steps.

QUESTIONS TO CONSIDER...REMEMBER, THERE IS A HUGE DIFFERENCE BETWEEN A FAST SURGEON AND AN EFFICIENT SURGEON

1. What am I doing to continually improve my surgical skills, decrease my operative times, decrease complications, and improve outcomes?

_____

_____

_____

_____

_____

_____

2. Am I continually going to conferences every year, and staying up to date on the advances in my subspecialty?

_____

_____

_____

_____

_____

_____

3. Can I take on tough cases and handle them well? If so, what can I do to get other surgeons in my community to send me cases?

_____

_____

_____

_____

_____

_____

4. Do I leverage industry relationships to do cadaver labs to improve my skills?

_____

_____

_____

_____

_____

_____

5. Do I have a network of surgeons to bounce complex cases off? What am I doing to continue to grow my network?

_____

_____

_____

_____

_____

6. Am I using an online database to track my outcomes?

_____

_____

_____

_____

_____

Chapter 7

Market Your Practice

If you truly want to expand your practice, then aside from establishing an efficient, smooth-running clinic, being an affable person, and performing excellent surgical work, you must prioritize your marketing efforts.

Liken the effort of starting your practice in a city to growing a forest. When you first arrive in your chosen metropolitan area, you have a barren landscape. Every new patient is a seed, and certain seeds are going to be planted and grow into trees, which then create more trees and more seeds, and so on and so on. Some of the most robust plants you'll grow will be the patients you successfully operate on; they will tell their friends and family about your practice and your referral base will grow. Traditionally, word-of-mouth has been the surest way to build a busy orthopedic practice.

That said, in the age of social media marketing, you must do more to stay competitive in the market. Patients prioritize word-of-mouth recommendations, but often they will check your website to find out more about you. They will consult your online reviews to confirm what they have heard from other people. If a patient hears from a friend that they had a great experience with you, yet they see few Google reviews online for you compared to another surgeon – or even worse, *poor* Google reviews – they will think twice about scheduling an appointment with you.

It always surprises me how frequently my patients tell me that they found me on the internet – a testament to our marketing efforts. Yes, you must have a great product and give a tremendous amount of value, and on the flip side, you must communicate that value to your community.

When we started in our group, we had eleven surgeons: nine older surgeons and two younger ones. As the younger surgeons amped up the marketing efforts, it became apparent that we had to hire a full-time marketer. It has been a huge boon to our practice. Prior that that, we depended on our administrators and MAs to set up meet-and-greets or dinners, or we hired outside marketing companies to promote us. It was an inefficient system. Based on my experience, the sooner you hire a marketer, the better.

Even in a small group of three- to- five surgeons, the starting salary for a marketer is around $60,000. If you utilize them appropriately, you will see a return on your investment the first year. It is a full-time job to set up meet and greets and dinners and allow you to showcase what you do in your practice. Your marketer can also handle your social media marketing, your website, and the 10,000 different little things that comprise a strategic marketing plan.

SEO, GMB, AND OTHER ASPECTS OF DIGITAL MARKETING

From a general marketing perspective, your website is vital. Research the various companies that develop medical websites. Whatever web development company you choose, ensure that your website facilitates easy patient feedback and funnels it into the different online review sites for each patient visit. This type of setup allows you to do what most companies do: provide a user-friendly method of receiving feedback from customers (patients) online. Most of your patients ought to be happy with their office visit and the quality of your work. The key is to make it simple for them to post about their experience and become an advocate for you. Our practices uses an excellent company called PatientPop.

It is also important to publish multiple videos on your website in which you introduce yourself, discuss the surgeries you perform, share what makes you unique, explain the different pathologies you treat, etc. Video testimonials from your patients are also powerful and provide social proof for potential patients who are viewing your website. Patients love videos, which make a much more profound impact than the written word. Remember, we are living in the YouTube era: the more videos on your site the better.

Be sure that the content on your website is easy to view on a smart-phone, and your website is smartphone-friendly since many people search the web that way. It is also vital to provide an easy-to-navigate online portal for patients to schedule appointments. Having one has been a huge benefit for us.

Making it easy for patients to schedule appointments with you extends beyond technology. A patient's interaction with your practice involves multiple factors; therefore, you must constantly work on the front desk, the schedulers that answer the phones, and the MAs that treat them. You are not the only person the patient deals with, so you cannot think solely of yourself. Every patient's sum experience with you is comprised of their interaction with your entire practice. Be sure that everyone on your staff provides excellent customer service.

In addition to developing an optimized website and managing your social media outreach, professional marketers can provide SEO, search engine optimization and other critical aspects of digital marketing like GMB, Google My Business (a moving target in an ever-changing tech environment). Hire professionals to do what they do best on your behalf; your job is to spend as much time as you can working with your patients and developing into an awesome surgeon.

I highly recommend a book called *Alignment: Strategic Research and Marketing Insights for the Thriving Orthopaedist,* written by Bill Champion, founder and president of Venel, an orthopedic consulting/marketing company. It is filled with useful information about how to market an orthopedic practice. If I could summarize the book's message in a few words, it is that we are in the people business, and an orthopedic surgeon's most effective marketing tool is to establish and maintain an excellent practice—meaning from the time the patient walks in the door until the time they leave, they have a wonderful experience. You must not only make it easy for patients to get in to see you, you must make it easy for referring docs to get their patients in to see you. It does not matter how good you are; if it is difficult for your peers to refer patients to you, they will stop doing it.

NEVER UNDERESTIMATE THE POWER OF IN-PERSON NETWORKING

Aside from hiring a professional digital marketing company, engage in another high-yield practice: hosting dinners with physicians or other referral sources such as chiropractors and physical therapists. In my experience, dinners with these healthcare professionals yield an excellent return on investment. As you share a meal, you can drill into their minds who you are and what you do. Of the three groups, doctors are often the most difficult to entice to dinner, but chiropractors and physical therapists have also proven to be an excellent source of referrals. One important caveat: you will have a much higher turnout if your guests believe they can get some referrals out of the dinner, too.

Regardless of your speciality, you must meet with these referral sources in a relaxed environment, where you can tell them more about you. In my group, I am the shoulder specialist; my partner is a hip, knee, and shoulder sports specialist; others are total joint surgeons; foot and ankle specialists, etc. When we sit down over dinner with our referral sources, we tell them what sets us apart in our respective specialties in a highly competitive field and city. We paint a picture in their minds of what we can offer to their patients. Our dinners take about an hour-and-a-half of our time yet generate a massive number of referrals.

Aside from meet-and-greets, lunches, and dinners, consider presenting at places like nursing homes and assisted living facilities. Yes, these activities can be exhausting, but if you truly desire to build and expand your practice, you must engage in them on a regular basis over a protracted period. Keep watering the seeds of your practice and watch it bloom beyond your wildest dreams.

A podiatrist friend of mine in town took this principle to an impressive level. When he first started his practice, he held meet-and-greets on Mondays, Wednesdays, and Fridays over lunch for three straight years. By the end of that period, he was seeing over 200 patients a week in his office – insane when you think about it. I'm not suggesting you host meet-a three days a week, but early on in your practice when you're not nearly as busy, dedicate one- to- two days a week to providing breakfast or lunch to primary care doctors. All you have to do is talk with them for a few minutes. It is more about interacting with their staff to ensure it is easy for them to refer patients to you. We use a form that features all the doctors in our office with checkboxes next to their names. Or you can give them your card and write your personal cell phone number on it. Seemingly simple things like that can make a huge difference.

In addition to finding new referral sources, make it a habit to follow up with the doctors and practices that already refer patients to get their feedback. You want to make sure they are happy because once a problem arises that causes them to stop sending patients your way it is too late. You must know if their patients are having a hard time getting in to see you or if any patients had a bad experience *before* they stop referring to you. If that happens, the game is over. Do not let small easy-to-fix problems turn into big, insurmountable obstacle. We visit our referring doctors on a regular basis to inquire if everything is going smoothly and address any issues they may have. We never ignore our core referral sources; we provide them and their patients with excellent service while we continue to build and grow.

Since orthopedic surgeons tend to avoid visiting other healthcare professionals' offices, use it to your advantage to set yourself apart from your surgeon-peers in your area. Early in my career when I applied this principle consistently, I discovered that these offices were taken aback that a surgeon planned to come in and provide lunch for them. They mistook me for a pharmaceutical rep because they were not accustomed to visits from orthopedic surgeons. The failure of most orthopedic surgeons to apply this marketing principle presents a golden opportunity for you to generate a steady stream of referrals.

SUCCESSFUL MARKETING BEGINS WITH YOU

Even though I have outlined several effective marketing strategies, none of them will work without a critical foundation: being an exceptional surgeon that treats patients like gold and delivers excellent outcomes. You cannot have a successful marketing campaign without a superior product or service, and in this case, that is YOU. Your brand as a surgeon is at the core of your marketing efforts, the sine qua non. Begin by following the principles I outlined in the chapters preceding this one and use strategic marketing to accelerate your natural progression.

Let us consider an example to illustrate my point. Two young surgeons we will call Surgeon A and Surgeon B are well-trained, skilled, and affable with their patients, who are happy with their services. Surgeon A makes it a priority to go out and meet primary doctors and host dinners every week. Surgeon A has also built an optimized website that features informative videos with patients, along with patient testimonial videos. Surgeon A's staff works like a well-oiled machine: they make it easy for patients to schedule their appointments and greet them warmly when they arrive at the office. With few exceptions, they work people into the schedule within one- to- two days – even when scheduling 50 patients a day. In addition, they make it a pleasure for primary care doctors and all other referral sources to send patients in to see them. Their website offers a mechanism that actively seeks feedback from all patients he sees, then pushes these reviews to the most high-yield patient review sites. The result? Surgeon A has an enviable amount of Google reviews. When patients search Surgeon A's practice online, he stands out as one of the highest rated and most reviewed doctors in the city.

On the other hand, Surgeon B, although just as qualified, skilled, and cordial as the first doctor, has a grouchy front desk and an MA that treats patients poorly. Early in his practice, he was so focused on getting through clinic and developing his surgical and clinical skills, he neglected to pay attention. His attitude about clinic was that it was just a means to an end – performing surgery, his first love. Yes, he knows the patient experience at his clinic is suffering because of his MA, but after a few years, he believes it would be too painful to let this person go. If he could travel backward in time, he would not have hired them; however, at this point he thinks it would demand too many hours and too much effort to train someone new to restore his train wreck of a clinic.

Furthermore, at least the current MA is "the devil he knows," whereas, a new hire would be an unknown quantity. He admits his clinic is inefficient with extended wait times that have nothing to do with him (or so he thinks). Surgeon B never goes out to meet primary care doctors because he is too busy – *he is an orthopedic surgeon for God's sake*! "It was painful enough to do that when I first got into practice," he thinks, "I am not putting myself through that awkwardness again." Sure, he wants to expand his practice, but he does not have time for things like dinner with other healthcare professionals. To compound his counterproductive attitude, his out-of-date website, designed by the cheapest vendor he could find, features scant information about him or his speciality...and zero videos. To make matters worse, it is almost impossible to access with a smartphone. Not surprisingly, there is no mechanism for patients to easily write and post a review, which is why Surgeon B has so few of them online. Yes, he has two or three 5-star reviews; however, that is not enough to provide social proof for potential new patients.

You see where I am going with this scenario. Even though at their core both surgeons provide excellent care, one of them neglects the "little things" outside of being an awesome surgeon. Hence, Surgeon A, who applies the marketing principles, expands his practice, and reaches his goals. It is a fact that one happy surgical patient tells 100 people about you for the rest of their life, while one unhappy patient moves the needle exponentially in the opposite direction. An effective marketing strategy begins with being an exceptional surgeon, then leveraging new technology, "old-fashioned" in-person networking, and word-of-mouth campaigns. Treat every patient like gold and accept every referral that comes your way.

EMBRACE THE DIFFICULT PATIENT

Here is a side note about marketing: you will see nutty patients in your practice, people who talk rudely to your staff and generally annoy everyone. You dread seeing them on the schedule, for understandable reasons. However, do your best to maintain objectivity and treat them the opposite of the way you think they deserve to be treated. I admit, I have had several patients that fit this category, where my MA just shakes her head and gives me that "look" as we pass each other on my way into the room. I think, "Oh no, this is going to be bad."

Many times, these patients have real problems that only you can resolve. If you can fix the crazy person and make them happy, you will become a god in their eyes. They will scream your name from the mountaintops till the end of time. Remember, some of your most difficult patients will make your practice unbelievably successful. They will refer 10,000 patients to you. It is challenging to deal with the crazy patient when you are in the middle of a busy clinic. You would much rather deal with the old farmer with a 2-cm rotator cuff tear, who has had an injection and has already done PT. You can just walk in, tell him he needs an operation to fix his problem, and hear him respond, "Yes, sir, whatever you think; you're the doctor and you know best."

These types of patients are easy on us, but if you can handle a difficult patient and solve their issue after they have already seen Surgeons X, Y, and Z – all of whom blew them off because they could not stand interacting with them, you will become so busy so freaking fast your head will spin.

CHAPTER 7 PRESCRIPTIONS FOR A HEALTHY PRACTICE

- ❖ In the age of social media marketing and advanced technology, you must do more than good surgery to stay competitive in the market.

- ❖ Make it easy for patients to schedule time with you.

- ❖ Hire a professional web designer to create an optimized website for your practice.

QUESTIONS TO CONSIDER...REMEMBER, IN THE DIGITAL AGE, YOU MUST LEVERAGE TECHNOLOGY TO BUILD A THRIVING PRACTICE

1. Do I have a full-time marketer? If not, what am I doing to get one?

_____

_____

_____

_____

_____

_____

2. Have I taken the time to review the content on my website? Are there multiple videos of me speaking? Patient testimonials? Information on my surgeries? Is my SEO optimized?

_____

_____

_____

_____

_____

_____

3. Is my website smartphone compatible?

_____

_____

_____

_____

_____

4. Do I have a system that allows me to actively seek reviews from my patients and then push those reviews to frequently visited patient review sites like Google and HealthGrades®, etc.?

_____

_____

_____

_____

_____

_____

5. Do I schedule regular dinners, lunches, or breakfasts to referring providers in my area?

_____

_____

_____

_____

_____

6. What am I doing to ensure it is easy for other physicians to refer patients to me? Do I communicate with them by sending them my notes for new patients and surgical?

_____

_____

_____

_____

_____

Chapter 8

Develop Other Income Streams

Why must surgeons develop other income streams? As I discussed in the chapter *Keep Your Sword Sharp*, thanks to an aging population, over the next 10 years we will be expected to perform an ever-increasing amount of surgery for less money. Becoming an efficient surgeon can help you alleviate and avoid any loss of income, but when you combine efficient surgery with the development of other income streams, you can achieve even greater financial prosperity. In this chapter, I will discuss two major income streams that have yielded a high return on my investment: ambulatory surgery centers (ASCs) and hospitals; and medical device companies.

Ambulatory Surgery Centers and Hospitals

Why invest in surgery centers? There are several reasons. First, coming out into private practice in the current healthcare market, most orthopedic surgeons need to supplement their income. For those who are employed by an academic institution, it is a different model but just about every private practicing orthopedist I know invests in at least one (and often multiple) surgery center. Therefore, it is imperative to understand the ins and outs of this income stream because knowledge is power.

Aside from income, another important motivation for orthopedic surgeons to own surgery centers is greater control over their operations. If you are a surgeon who works at a hospital, you are at the whims of the hospital CEO and management. They establish the protocols, dictate the hospital set-up and design, and control its management. They also tell you what implants you can purchase. Whereas when you own your surgery center, you have complete control of everything from the staffing to the entire setup. Essentially, you are the boss. That allows you to create and maintain a streamlined operation in which you can establish efficiency, hire the best people, and entrust your most exceptional employees with the management of your center.

In addition, surgery centers offer physicians much more control over where they perform surgery. Time and time again, it has been shown that physician-owned facilities outperform non-physician-owned facilities on multiple levels including cost, quality, and outcomes. In the future, the quality of healthcare will improve because physician-owned facilities give physicians direct control over the treatment and management of patients.

Now let us look at the income potential of this second revenue stream. When you analyze the overall cost of a surgery, most of it comes from the facility. For instance, if you perform a rotator cuff repair, you may receive $2,000- to- $3,000 from most insurance companies or Medicare. Your anesthesiologist may receive around $500, but the facility will receive anywhere from $5,000- to- $12,000, with different insurance contracts. That means most of the healthcare costs associated with surgery are tied up with the facility. By owning a percentage of a facility, if you can create a scenario in which your income exceeds your overhead, you make a profit. Therefore, owning surgery centers provides a method for surgeons to generate a second revenue stream outside of doing surgery. It is not necessarily a *passive* revenue stream; it is *pseudo* passive in the sense that you must have active players involved to generate the income.

For many of the surgeons in my group, investing in surgery centers is an excellent source of additional income. They generate more revenue from their investments in surgery centers and surgical hospitals than they do for being surgeons, which can be good and bad. But before you invest in a surgery center or surgical hospital, you must understand the rules and laws governing them. While I am no expert on the law, I will share a brief synopsis of what I have learned in my short time in practice.

Over the past 25 years, there has been an explosion of ambulatory surgery centers (ACS), much of it due to an increase in outpatient surgery. When you look at surgery 30- to- 40 years ago, fewer were performed, and when surgeons did operate on patients, they kept them in the hospital for longer periods of time. Today, with the prevalence of outpatient surgery, that has shifted. If you had informed surgeons back in the mid-70s or early 80s that the trend in healthcare was outpatient surgery and that orthopedic doctors would perform a significant amount of total knees and total hips as outpatients, they would have thought you were crazy.

But techniques have evolved. Our implants, pain control, and anesthesia have improved to such an extent that outpatient surgery will be the standard in the future. In fact, you will be forced to make a compelling case for performing these types of surgeries in a traditional hospital. This significant shift in the number of outpatient surgeries versus inpatient surgeries creates opportunities for investment in small surgery centers.

Decreased physician reimbursements are another factor in the decision to invest in surgery centers. Psychologically, as human beings, when something is taken away from us, we focus our efforts on holding our ground instead of growing and building. For surgeons in the 1980s, overall reimbursements were much better. But when they started to decrease in the 90s for many procedures, physicians started to examine ways to leverage themselves within the system. Owning their own facility was a great way to do that. Today, for a doctor coming out in practice, it is unusual *not* to have some sort of ownership, given the history of reimbursements. That is why you must understand the distinction between a hospital and a surgery center. A hospital is a place where you do inpatient and outpatient surgery whereas an ASC is for outpatient surgery only, though some of them have 23-hour observation rooms. But the main distinction between a hospital and an ASC involves Medicare and the ability to do surgeries for which Medicare requires an inpatient stay. If you are going to do a total shoulder or a total hip procedure on a Medicare patient, at present you must do it in an inpatient hospital because there is no outpatient code. They recently changed the rules to allow you to do total knees as an outpatient, but total shoulders and total hips still require an inpatient stay. For these procedures, you need beds and the ability to keep patients overnight.

THE AFFORDABLE CARE ACT, ANTI-KICKBACK STATUTE, STARK LAW AND THEIR EFFECT ON ASCs

The passage of the Affordable Care Act in 2010 placed a hold or a lockdown on any new physician-owned hospitals that accepted Medicare. Prior to 2010, you could build a hospital with a group of doctors for various reasons. But the Affordable Care Act drew a line in the sand and told doctors who owned hospitals that they could no longer bill Medicare, although they could still build hospitals. However, since Medicare comprises a significant amount of a hospital's reimbursement, it does not make sense to build one. On the other hand, the Affordable Care Act did not place any type of moratorium on ASC's and, as a result, they have exploded over the past 10 years.

Most of the laws governing hospitals and surgery centers originate with the Anti-Kickback Statute and Stark Law. For a deeper understanding, I suggest researching them or consulting with a healthcare lawyer. My purpose here is to share the experience and knowledge I accrued from being in practice. Anti-Kickback Laws and Stark Law revolve around not being able to pay surgeons to do surgery at certain centers, meaning, you cannot offer them direct payments as incentive to do surgery. You cannot give it and you cannot take it away. If a surgeon is doing surgery at a facility where they have a percent ownership, and they cut down their volume, the center cannot tell them, "Oh, we're going to take away X amount of your shares because you brought in less volume." On the other hand, they cannot do the opposite by promising surgeons, "If you do X number of cases, we will sell you X percentage of shares."

That said, there are some ways you can structure your arrangement to ensure your surgeons are performing surgeries. Otherwise, the entity ceases to exist, right? Like any other business, a surgery center must bring in revenue – and that revenue comes from surgeries. If an ASC's surgeons are not performing enough surgeries, it will not be profitable. Therefore, your surgeons must be invested in it both monetarily and in terms of their cases. If your investment in your ASC is to yield a healthy return, you must understand the metrics.

Let us say you are an owner in an ASC, and you want to bring on a new partner. Establish a vetting period of three- to- six months during which they perform surgeries because it is vital to confirm their excellence as a surgeon, their ability to bring in a certain amount of volume, and their attitude toward your staff. This vetting period should help you develop trust that you can give them a percentage of ownership in your facility in exchange for significant patient volume. You can decide that volume on the front end; you just cannot take anything away on the back end. Even though you cannot directly incentivize people, you can indirectly incentivize them.

The trouble comes after someone gets their hands on the shares after they have stopped doing cases or are doing the bare minimum of cases, yet still taking large payments. This scenario plays out in centers across America: in the early stages, a surgeon does high volume, or was one of the initial investors before the center was built – precluding an opportunity to vet them – only to stop contributing to the overall success of the ASC.

If you choose to get involved with a group of surgeons in an ASC and simply accept handshake agreements on each person's responsibilities, make sure you can trust them. You cannot create a written contract that clearly states they must do X number of cases or else get kicked out. That is illegal. Therefore, trust your instincts, do your research, and select partners who will work as hard as you do. Ensure that, number one, they are busy; and number two, they will honor their commitment regarding the number of cases they will bring to the ASC. It is a good idea to ask them to a sign a document that confirms the number of cases they do per year and any other centers they are already invested in to make sure they do not spread themselves too thin. Oftentimes, a group of surgeon-investors will invest in a new surgery center, then over time, invest in another facility as their practice starts to wind down. They stop bringing cases to the ASC, yet they maintain a large ownership in the facility, and still receive a large monthly or bimonthly distribution check. In these situations, it is extremely difficult to take their shares away from them. That is why you must exercise caution and put serious thought into choosing your co-investors.

IF YOU (OR YOUR DEVELOPER) BUILD IT, THEY WILL COME

As Kevin Costner famously stated in the movie, *Field of Dreams*, "if you build it, they will come." When it comes to surgery centers, however, busy surgeons do not necessarily have to build them themselves. It is difficult to take time out of our day to physically erect a building, hire the nurses and the rest of the staff, and navigate the regulatory processes necessary to get a surgery center up and running. Yes, some surgeons take on these responsibilities themselves, much to their benefit. However, if you do not have the time or the inclination to handle it all yourself, there are multiple management companies out there that can help you. A few you might have heard of include Amsurg, United Surgical Partners International (USPI), Surgical Care Affiliates (SCA), and Surgical Center Development, Inc. (SCDI). These management companies build out the center; help you take out loans; assemble groups of surgeon-investors for the property; hire all the staff; manage all the operations; and build the center. In a nutshell, you hire them to run the center for you. They get a percent of ownership in the facility, much like a partner, so if the center becomes profitable, they become profitable. If the center is not profitable, they are not profitable. Most of these centers generate significant profits if they are full of busy surgeons performing multiple surgeries.

The other partnership we commonly see with hospitals has less to do with management and more to do with insurance contracts – leveraging and contracting with insurance companies. The more leverage you have over the insurance company in terms of billing volume, the better your contracts. That is why big hospital systems, though inefficient, have tremendous leverage over insurance companies. If the hospitals go out of network on that insurance company, they will take a hit since the hospital system enjoys a large share of the patient market. Therefore, everything is about leverage. To get the best insurance contracts, you must partner with the hospitals. It is as simple as that.

Sometimes you will notice dual partnerships where a surgery center management company is invested in the center. They help build it, run it, and manage the day-to-day operations. Second are the physician partners, and third, a hospital partner. The hospital partner's role is to provide the insurance contracts; in return, they receive a percent ownership of the facility. The more players involved, the more watered down the revenue. You want to strike the right balance to ensure a good return on your investment. Still, this arrangement in which a hospital (along with a management company and a group of physicians) owns a percentage of the facility is quite common.

You might wonder how these types of centers generate profit. It is simple. When you perform surgery at a surgery center, you will receive payments from insurance companies. You can also receive cash pay, but most of your income will originate from insurance companies and Medicare. Of course, you must pay for your overhead. What is the overhead at a surgery center? Well, you must pay the people that work there:

nurses, technicians, cleaning crew, administrators, etc. In addition, you must pay for all your leases because often these surgery centers are in leased spaces. On the front end, there is a build-out period where you must pay for the facility to be outfitted with all the equipment you need to do surgery. That is your responsibility.

Many physicians take out a loan to pay for these required front-end expenses. Not only do you have the monthly lease payment of the property, you have your loan payments from procuring the necessary items and build-out to customize it for surgery. For a specific period, that is a fixed cost. The biggest controllable cost is your implants. When we perform orthopedic surgery at these facilities, we use implants and equipment that comprise a huge chunk of overhead. Once you account for all these costs, if you run the center efficiently by keeping costs down and the surgery volume high, you will generate a profit.

Are some surgery centers unprofitable? Yes, some yield zero or even negative profit. On the opposite end of the spectrum, there are some centers where invested surgeons make over seven figures in profit. And then there is everything in between. It all comes down to the surgical volume and how lucrative the contracts are. What is the revenue coming in from their surgeries and what are their costs? A thriving center with top-notch contracts can be extremely profitable. If it is a surgeon-owned hospital, it can be even more profitable.

There are multiple factors that determine the success or failure of a surgery center, but the most important one pertains to the doctors and the surgeries. If you have a group of hard-working, busy surgeons, your surgery center will see a profit every month; however, if you have a group of mediocre surgeons or surgeons that bring in minimal volume – or volume that is well below what they promised – the center will not be profitable. You must think about this in terms of the metrics and the numbers, with the understanding that overhead expenses are fixed.

For instance, let us say the monthly overhead at a two-room input ambulatory surgery center is $300,000. That means to break even and keep the facility open, you must generate over $300,000 in revenue. It keeps the building open and pays the nurses, the staff, and all the fixed expenses. Everything after that is profit. You must ask yourself, "What do we need to do to achieve that number, and how far beyond that number can we get with our current group?" First, you must reach a certain break-even point, and it takes time to build up a center's volume. But once you get it going, it can generate an excellent profit.

Another way to generate profit from surgery centers is to sell portions of it. Here is a common scenario: a group of surgeons build an ambulatory surgery center, nurture it for five years, turn it into an exceptionally profitable venture in which they generate high volume and ROI, and then sell a portion of it to a hospital system with better contracts. They always do this at specific times in the earning cycle. Let us suppose the earnings of your center was a million dollars. You will sell it to the hospital for five times that amount, or $5 million. In return, you will get a better contract. If you can build a center from the ground up and make it profitable, just like any other company, you can sell it – or a portion of it – to a bigger company or sell a portion of it to a bigger company, e.g. a hospital. You get better contracts; they get a percentage of ownership. It is a win-win in which you walk away with a sizable check but keep a percentage of ownership.

When evaluating a surgery center or company, there are specific questions you must ask before you invest. Your decision may be determined when you join your orthopedic group because many groups own their own centers or large portions of centers, giving you an opportunity to buy into it as an investment. Regardless, you must ask the following questions:

➤ How long has it been open?

➤ How much debt does it have?

➤ Have they paid off their initial loan?

➤ What did it cost to build out the space?

➤ What are the fixed expenses?

➤ What is the overhead?

➤ What is the profit? How long has the facility generated it?

➤ What is the maximum percent ownership I can have in the surgery center, per the operating agreement and what is the cost?

➤ How many surgeons are invested and what percent ownership does each have?

Analyze the numbers just as you would for any business and ask for simple terms because they will give you a bunch of spreadsheets with 10,000 items on them. Stick to the questions above. In terms of maximum percent ownership, with some facilities it is one- to- two percent; others go as high as 10 percent. Then, there is everything in between. You want to find out the maximum percent you can own. Note it as a percentage – do not get caught up in the number of shares. I speak from experience because I made that mistake early on. For me, it was always about shares. Well, shares are arbitrary, but a percent ownership is set. You could have 10,000 shares at one facility and 100 shares at another facility. The number of shares they create is a moving target, and sometimes centers will create more shares, which dilutes the ownership.

Again, you must ask, "What percent ownership do I have?" It is a simple equation: you have a percent ownership of a facility that generates a profit every year, so just do the math. Whatever percent you own, in most centers you receive a percentage of those profits. If you think about it in these terms, percent ownership and how much it costs you, it will be much easier for your brain to grasp. However, inquire also about the typical distribution. For example, if you own X percent, how much is it going to generate in distributions? How much is that going to cost?

Often, they will give you this information in a cost-per-share. The share may cost $1,000 and generate a profit each year of $500. You as a surgeon can come in and buy 10 shares for $10,000 and expect to see a profit/distribution of $5,000. Here are two random examples. In a physician-owned hospital, the shares can be expensive. Often the share price is determined by a multiple of the share. And that multiple is determined by the profitability of the center and how long it has been open. Some companies come in simply to evaluate the shares. They analyze the health of the center: How many cases are they doing? How long have they been profitable? How long have they been open? What is the mix of surgeons? What are the trends? These are the factors they consider in their valuation, which can be anywhere from two times the value at the low end, up to seven to eight times. Let us assume a share distributes $3,000 a year. If it is a healthy center or surgical hospital that has been open for a decade and generating profit for a significant amount of time, the shares will be expensive.

The share price could range anywhere from $15,000 to $20,000 per share. When you examine the numbers, you think, "Wow, these places can be expensive to invest in." Whereas, when you consider a brand-new surgery center starting from the ground up, you can get seven- to-eight percent ownership of that facility for $50,000. Think of it in terms of buying stock in Coca Cola or Apple, versus investing in a start-up company. Coca Cola is a 100-year-old company that has turned a profit for a long time. Apple is another established and profitable brand – as opposed to a start-up tech company. If you get involved with the right surgeons, surgery centers are not quite as risky as tech companies; however, they still come with the risk that the other investing surgeons will not live up to their promises. In this case, you can get a large percentage of ownership for a small amount of money, but your risk is greater because you have no idea how it is going to play out with the surgeons.

If you align with a trustworthy group of people who live up to their commitment in terms of cases, it can be unbelievably profitable. It is one of the best investments you can ever make with your time and money. But I have learned my lesson the hard way that you cannot trust everybody's word about the cases they will bring to the center. I cannot stress enough the importance of not only evaluating the center, but even more critically, the surgeons that operate there. If a center is already up and running, to evaluate its health, focus on its current volume, the percent ownerships of the various surgeons, and their case volume. If a large percentage of the center's distributions go to surgeons that do not perform surgery, it is an unhealthy center. If the center has a bunch of younger surgeons (who tend to generate more volume) that do not have a significant percentage in the center, it is an unhealthy center.

Finally, review the non compete. If you are considering getting involved in two different facilities, this is crucial information to have. Look at the non compete on the front end and protect yourself on the back end. These are some of the most important things I can think of.

Overall, investing in a surgery center can be an amazing opportunity to control your own destiny in terms of its operations and to provide incredible, high-quality care. It is the way of the future for sure. However, when you consider investing in surgery centers, especially when you are just coming out in practice, it is up to you to do your due diligence. Evaluate the center and align yourself with the proper management companies and the right surgeons.

CONSULT WITH MEDICAL DEVICE COMPANIES

Coming into a new practice, another excellent way to develop name-recognition in your speciality, market yourself, and generate more revenue by leveraging the system is to consult with medical device companies. Your ability to generate revenue here is twofold. One, you will get paid for your time. If you get a contract as a consultant you can teach courses, conferences, and advise medical device companies on product development. They will pay you an hourly rate that varies from company to company and from surgeon to surgeon. In my experience, it falls between a minimum of $400 and a maximum of $800. Some of the Anti Kickback Laws and regulations around this were established about six years ago. The government tried to limit exorbitant payments for orthopedic physicians for medical device consulting. Consequently, you cannot make $10,000 to go to a conference for an hour; your earnings must be in alignment with the general salary of a working orthopedist, but you will get paid for your time.

Second, if you help with the development of a product, you will often receive a percent royalty, which also varies. At the low end, it can be less than one percent and go as high as five percent or more, depending on the relationship with the company and how many surgeons are involved with the project. This is a great opportunity for a young orthopedist to create another revenue stream – and more importantly, develop relationships. Often, when you become a consultant for a company, you get to teach courses, travel to the company headquarters, and interact with other surgeons – typically, the most prominent leaders in our field.

When you attend industry-sponsored meetings, you can learn from the best. Yes, you are the one teaching but you will also learn and network with the busiest and most exceptional surgeons. It is an excellent way to develop relationships with industry partners. You can get an insider look at how these companies work, what products they have in development, and what is coming down the pipe.

Via my involvement with device manufacturing companies, I have learned a lot about the business side, how products, are developed, and what goes into bringing a product to the market. More valuable, by attending and teaching with other surgeons at these industry-led conferences, I have learned more about surgery and becoming a better orthopedist. Although medical device companies use these events to drive sales, they know the best way to do that is to provide an excellent educational forum for surgeons. It is not just to market their products but to help surgeons hone their skills and perform higher quality surgery while utilizing their product. Conferences are a wonderful opportunity to develop beneficial relationships on both sides. Remember, though, you always get paid for your time when you are a consultant.

And then the real path to passive revenue is to induce device manufacturing companies put you on projects and give you a royalty on product sales. That said, when you look at the CMS open payment data, you will note that many surgeons who make large royalties from these companies have been with them for five- to- 10 years. Look at it from the company's standpoint: if they make you a part of the development team for a product, they want to know that the relationship will be long lasting. You cannot bounce back and forth between companies and expect to be put on meaningful projects.

Furthermore, medical device companies do not like surgeons that want to be on the front end or are aggressive about asking for payment for their services. They want to see that you are going to be a good partner for the long haul; someone they can trust as a leader in their field who will help them expand their sales base. The bottom line is that they are trying to sell more products. And they want to know that you are not just angling for a royalty check or consulting payments but want to partner with them for years to come. When you speak with the decision-makers in these companies, remember they are looking for a creative and innovative surgeon;

one who gets along well with people, does not have an oversized ego, and wants to assist the company in expanding their portfolio.

Medical device manufacturing companies are seeking effective ambassadors for them and their products. Therefore, be genuine. If you do not believe in a company or their products, do not teach comprehensive courses about them. Get involved with a company that manufactures high-quality products and provides tremendous value to orthopedic surgeons and their patients.

When you are new in practice, the best way to initiate a relationship with a medical device company is to strike up a conversation with the local reps in your area. Let them know, "Hey, I want to be involved. I want to teach, and I want to work with your company." Select one or two companies whose products you use the most. Do not get involved in too many because it will become stressful and overwhelming. Once you express interest, they will fly you in to discuss the path you must follow with their company. And the best way to determine the path of progress is to talk to surgeons that have been consulting with them for five, 10, or 15 years. So long as you are a specialist and a leader, the company will find a way to get you involved. Then it is off to the races.

You royalty potential in this scenario is sky high. However, it takes a significant amount of work on the front end. If you have amazing ideas for awesome products and present them to the medical device company, you will earn royalties much quicker, but remember, you are utilizing their infrastructure, engineers, and leverage to bring that product to market; therefore, you will own much less of it than if you had started your own company. Now, it is much less risky because it involves less of your capital and a smaller investment of your time, energy, and money. Yes, it generates less revenue. However, many surgeons have created a nice income stream by getting products to market in conjunction with existing companies.

Keep in mind, it is not just about a great product; it must be something that fits in well with their portfolio. It must make sense for them to financially to develop it. If they do not feel the current market justifies the intensive and costly process of bringing your product to market, they will not do it. Their decision hinges not solely on a fabulous idea but whether the idea will make the company money. These companies must turn a profit; otherwise, they will cease to exist. They satisfy a need for medical devices to perform the surgeries we must do for our patients. The bigger companies tend to move a slower than the smaller companies, but they also have deeper pockets and a much larger sales force. Even though you get a smaller percentage of the royalty, your ceiling is expansive. In the beginning, it probably makes the most sense to align with an existing company to take your idea from concept to reality.

Of course, you may hit a roadblock. If you still think it is a great product and you want to bring it to market, you can always do it yourself – which requires a whole other book on the subject. The number one benefit I have found when doing the device consulting is learning from the other surgeons that teach with me at conferences and developing relationships with leaders in the field, many of whom are also the high-end consultants. I have learned much about the inner workings of medical device companies and the orthopedic market. On the back end, I have gotten some revenue from it. Remember you will not make any more from this than you would from seeing more patients and doing more surgery; depending on how busy your surgery schedule is, you may even make less. A simple way to determine if it is worth your time is to review the amount of time you spend in surgery. Add up the hours and see how much you make from all your surgical and clinical collections. Do the math. If the math reveals you make $500 per hour or $1,000 per hour, review your consulting contract.

If you figure out, "I'm not really making any more by doing this. It is typically a wash," or "I *lose* a little money by doing the consulting," you are not consulting to generate more money, because you can make more money just working on your practice. The ultimate benefit of consulting comes from learning and developing relationships. And if your goal is to help innovate and create new products and leverage it with a royalty from a company, you must remember that it happens on the back end over time. It requires patience because many physicians are already working with medical device companies on these things, which means you must get in line behind much more prominent surgeons that have been practicing for 10, 15, or 20 years. That said, I know some high-producing young surgeons that have excellent relationships with medical device companies. These companies know they will innovate and lead the field for years to come. Within my first five to 10 years of practice, we got lucrative agreements. It is a path to creating passive revenue, while remaining aligned with your values as a surgeon. Again, to get started, engage in a conversation with the medical device reps. That will lead to upper level management flying you to their headquarters, where you can discuss your goals and map out a strategy for achieving them.

CHAPTER 8 PRESCRIPTIONS FOR A HEALTHY PRACTICE

- ❖ Make it a priority to develop other income streams.

- ❖ Consider with care the surgeons you choose to align with in a surgery center or hospital.

- ❖ Ask the right questions before you commit to any arrangement with a surgery center or hospital.

- ❖ Initiate conversations with your medical device reps to receive an invitation to company headquarters to discuss your goals.

- ❖ Use the opportunity when teaching courses with other surgeons to learn, network, and nurture beneficial relationships.

QUESTIONS TO CONSIDER...REMEMBER, CHOOSE YOUR OPPORTUNITIES AND SURGEONS WISELY

1. What steps am I taking to develop other income streams?

_____

_____

_____

_____

_____

_____

2. Have I researched opportunities to invest in an ASC? Why or why not?

_____

_____

_____

_____

_____

3. Do I network with enough orthopedic surgeons to identify potential partners for an ASC or physician-owned hospital?

_____

_____

_____

_____

_____

_____

4. Have I narrowed down my choices to two medical device companies?

_____

_____

_____

_____

_____

5. What have I done to initiate relationships with my medical device reps?

_____

_____

_____

_____

_____

_____

6. Am I willing to travel to conferences, teach with other surgeons, network, and follow the prescribed path the medical device companies lay out for me?

_____

_____

_____

_____

_____

_____

7. Can I commit to partnering with these companies for at least five years?

_____

_____

_____

_____

_____

_____

Chapter 9

Maintain a Healthy Quality of Life

When I put this book together, my main goal was to share the 9 core *Dr. Hustle* principles I have applied to build a thriving, successful practice. However, the first eight principles will do little good if you do not first get in touch with your "why." Why did you become an orthopedic surgeon in the first place? It is a given that most of us are driven, Type-A personalities; otherwise, we would not have chosen surgery as a career path. But what is your underlying motivation?

Remember, life is a marathon, not a sprint. Years from now, when you look back on your life, will you focus solely on what you accomplished as an orthopedic surgeon? Or will you reflect upon the kind of citizen, neighbor, spouse, parent, friend, sister, brother, son, or daughter you were? How would you like to feel about the quality of your relationships and the experiences you had outside of work?

As a husband and father, I know how difficult it can be to strike the right balance and maintain a healthy quality of life. When I sat down to write this book, it did not occur to me to write about this topic until another busy orthopedic friend suggested it. That is when I realized my book would be incomplete without a discussion of work-life-family balance. Isn't that why we all want to get home sooner rather then later? Establishing and maintaining an efficient practice and operating room brimming with patients not only makes you more successful from a professional standpoint, it frees up time for your personal priorities – whether they involve a spouse and children, a game of golf, travel, or an enjoyable hobby. Whatever your motivation for wanting to get home as quickly as possible, I encourage you to apply the 9 core principles in this book to shave an hour or two off your clinic day (while seeing more patients) and shave off an hour or two off your operating day (while performing more surgery).

Authors Clay M. Christensen, James Allworth, and Karen Dillon wrote an excellent book on this subject entitled, *How Will You Measure Your Life?* (A highly intelligent guy, I recommend that you read Christensen's other books, too.) It reflects upon his life and the lives of some successful businesspeople he trained during his tenure as a professor at Harvard Business School. According to Christensen, these folks were unbelievably successful professionals, but they had disastrous personal lives, characterized by multiple divorces and poor relationships with their children.

He wondered why this was so, and in his book, he breaks it down into solid points. Most of these professionals did not notice the damage caused by their failure to focus on their spouse and children until it was too late. They stayed an extra hour at work, took on an additional meeting, missed their daughter's recital or their son's big game, or forgot about date night with their spouse. Even when they were home, they were not present; instead, they let their phones, emails, and other work-related items distract them.

In this sense, they are like other driven professionals in various fields. You can get away with this behavior for a long time without seeing the wreckage it inflicts on your personal relationships – much like smoking, overeating, or many of the habits we counsel our patients to avoid. And, like cancer, it can be insidious. If you are a smoker, by the time you realize you have stage four lung cancer, it is too late. On a relationship level, by the time your husband or wife serves you the divorce papers, the relationship has reached the point of no return. And if your kids are in their teens or young adults when you finally decide you have neglected them for too long and want to spend more time with them, chances are it will be too late to restore these relationships.

The problem for orthopedic surgeons is that you must invest time in your career on the front end; but if you make that your life focus while ignoring your family, friends, and quality of life, on the back end you will realize you made a huge mistake. If you can recognize and learn the lesson now, you can avoid this unwanted outcome. Christensen's book made me realize that I must continually force myself to redirect my focus to ensure all aspects of my life are in balance.

Another set of great books I highly recommend come from Stephen Covey, an author best known for, *The 7 Habits of Highly Effective People*. However, Covey's *The 8th Habit: From Effectiveness to Greatness* has made the most profound impact on my life. It talks about not only improving your efficiency and effectiveness at work, ensuring that your energy and focus are on the aspects of your life that align with your core values as a human being.

It is pretty rare for any professional to deny that they want to be a great spouse or parent; however, for surgeons in particular, it is easy to let our work overwhelm us to the point where our personal relationships take a back seat to our careers. Our spouse and our children become the second or third thing, instead of the first thing. One of Covey's most effective analogies (watch a video demonstration of this principle from one of his conferences on YouTube) involves putting rocks in a jar.

In your life, the rocks represent the most important things. For many of us, that means our spouse and children; for others, it could be our parents, friends, or hobbies. Other rocks can include spirituality. Take the big rocks in your life and place them in the jar first. Next, add the smaller rocks – the meetings, conferences, research papers, and all the other things that go along with your career. These smaller rocks fit in around the larger rocks. Next, fill the cracks with sand that represents the little things in life. Lastly, fill the jar with water – all the little nonsensical things we do, the business-of-life details.

If you put the big rocks in first, all the other stuff will fill in the cracks. But if you fill everything in with pebbles and sand, you will not have room for the big rocks. I love thinking about life this way because it clarifies everything so well. You must put the big rocks in first – make time for your family, and when you do, turn off your phone and your computer. You would not dream of missing a clinic or a surgery, and this is no different. Show up for your family with the same amount of discipline and commitment you apply to your profession. Once your workday is over and you stop booking surgeries, leave your clinic not just physically, but mentally, so you can spend quality time with the ones you love.

When I was in my first year of practice, I heard another motivating talk at the Arthroscopy Association, given by a busy shoulder surgeon named JT Tokish. A U.S. military veteran, he served overseas for several years. This intelligent, active guy also publishes multiple papers. If you have not yet met him, I hope you do soon because he is an outstanding person. During his presentation, he pulled many surgeons from his former fellowship that had been in practice anywhere from two- to- 25 years, for the purpose of discovering their level of satisfaction with their lives. It turned out the only factor that they associated with happiness was how much they worked.

What do they do outside of work? Spend time with their spouse and children, engage in their favorite hobbies, attend cultural and sporting events, exercise, and in general, enjoy life outside of the clinic and OR. Because what is the point of working 80- to- 90 hours a week to become successful and make a lot of money, only to feel unfulfilled? If the rest of your life is out of balance, nothing else matters. That is why you must constantly ask yourself, "What are my priorities?" and "What are my values?" Write them down. Then, find the discipline to say NO to the unimportant stuff.

My purpose in writing this book is to help you build a busy and efficient practice that enables you to generate your desired income in half the time. If my readers apply the 9 core principles that I have outlined to achieve their professional and personal goals, that would be a dream come true for me. Even if just one person absorbs and applies these lessons gleaned from experience, it will have been worth the effort.

I look forward to receiving emails and phone calls saying something like, *"I saw more patients today in less time and still provided excellent quality of care. I perform more surgeries now, too. And we all go home sooner. I see my wife and kids more and I am making more money that I have ever made despite having more quality time for myself and my family. Life is great!"*

That is the ultimate right there. It is a win-win on multiple levels. Again, the key is to set your priorities, schedule your times, and then stick to them. Put the big rocks in the jar first; once you do that, everything else will fill in. Remember to take quality time to rest and refresh your system. When I played football in high school and college, I worked out all the time. But I soon learned about a phenomenon known as over-training: when you lift weights too often, the body breaks down, resulting in overuse injuries. Then, you move backwards instead of forward because you are not getting stronger.

If you want to get stronger, you must alternate stressing and resting the system. Yes, you want to constantly push the limits of what you can do as an orthopedist, but you also need time to back off, rest, and allow your mind and brain to reset. You can do this by playing a round of golf, running, or biking through a park, riding your motorcycle, or whipping up a gourmet meal in the kitchen. Whatever it is, give yourself the gift of indulging in activities that uplift, inspire, and allow you to decompress.

In the book, *Peak Performance: Elevate Your Game, Avoid Burnout, and Thrive with the New Science of Success,* authors Brad Stulberg and Steve Magness explain that professional, phenomenal athletes push themselves to the limit when they train, but then back off to rest. They feed their bodies proper nutrition and get adequate sleep. In our demanding profession, it is imperative that we take care of our bodies and our minds by eating right and getting good quality sleep every night. You must do things outside of medicine to keep yourself balanced and energized. When you do, you will become a better physician.

You also need to exercise. It is easy to get sucked into a mentality that you are just too busy or do not have the time to exercise as much as you should. Yet exercise adds juice to the battery. It increases your capacity to work because it improves your energy and focus, which makes everything in your life better. Eat a healthy diet, exercise on a regular basis, and go to bed on time. These three practices will make a huge impact on your quality of life. As with your relationships, if you fail to eat right, exercise, and sleep by the time you realize the error of your ways, it will be too late. Prioritize good nutrition, proper exercise, and quality sleep now...and watch your life transform into something beautiful.

We orthopedic surgeons have worked too hard for too long not to take time off for ourselves and our loved ones. Protect the people and things that matter most to you, just as you protect your surgery and clinic time. All of us show up every single day for clinic and surgery; we would never, ever miss those things. Apply the same discipline to other facets of your life and avoid waking up one day in the future, filled with regrets.

In my practice, I do not work on Fridays or on the weekends. I have not taken ER calls since my first year in practice. These decisions have helped me maintain a healthy work-life balance. I am still evolving in my efforts to carve out time for my family and to play golf and do some of the other things that make me a well-rounded, balanced person but I have made significant progress.

I hope I have demonstrated through these 9 core principles that you can manifest an abundant income as a busy, efficient orthopedic surgeon *and* enjoy a high-quality, balanced life filled with the people and things that bring you joy. You do not have to choose between one or the other; it is all about setting your priorities and creating efficiencies.

Whether you are happily single or happily married, you deserve to lead a fulfilling life if you want to excel in your career as an orthopedic surgeon for years to come. It simply requires you to focus your energy on your personal relationships and your physical, mental, and spiritual wellbeing …before it is too late.

CHAPTER 9 PRESCRIPTIONS FOR A HEALTHY PRACTICE

❖ Reflect upon your "why."

❖ Put the big rocks in the jar first; then everything else will fill in.

❖ Read motivational books from Clay M. Christensen and Steven Covey.

❖ When you leave the clinic or the OR for the day, check out mentally as well as physically so you can be fully present with the most important people in your life.

❖ Remember the goal is to establish an efficient practice so you can earn more money in less time and free up more time for your loved ones, and to refresh your body, mind, and spirit by engaging in activities that bring you the most joy.

QUESTIONS TO CONSIDER...REMEMBER, A LIFE WELL-LIVED ENCOMPASSES SO MUCH MORE THAN A SUCCESSFUL CAREER

1. What motivated me to become an orthopedic surgeon?

_____

_____

_____

_____

_____

_____

2. What are my goals and priorities outside of work?

_____

_____

_____

_____

_____

3. What activities bring me the most joy?

_____

_____

_____

_____

_____

4. Do I make time to exercise?

_____

_____

_____

_____

_____

5. Am I getting adequate sleep every night?

_____

_____

_____

_____

_____

6. Do I consume a healthy diet?

_____

_____

_____

_____

_____

7. Are my personal relationships fulfilling? If not, what can I do to improve them?

_____

_____

_____

_____

_____

References

Patient Pop

https://www.patientpop.com/

A Roadmap for New Physicians: Fraud and Abuse Laws

https://oig.hhs.gov/compliance/physician-education/01laws.asp

Stark Law

https://en.wikipedia.org/wiki/Stark_Law#:~:text=Stark%20Law%20is%20a%20set,a%20financial%20relationship%20with%20that

Affordable Care Act

https://www.healthcare.gov/glossary/affordable-care-act/

Alignment: Strategic Research and Marketing Insights for the Thriving Orthopaedist

https://www.amazon.com/Alignment-Strategic-Research-Marketing-Orthopaedist/dp/160544040X

Venel

https://www.venel.com/#home

The 7 Habits of Highly Effective People, Stephen R. Covey

The 8th Habit: From Effectiveness to Greatness, Stephen R. Covey

Peak Performance: Elevate Your Game, Avoid Burnout, and Thrive with the New Science of Success, Brad Stulberg, Steve Magness

How Will You Measure Your Life?, Clayton M. Christensen, James Allworth, Karen Dillon

Physician-Owned Surgical Hospitals Outperform Other Hospitals in Medicare Value-Based Purchasing Program

Google My Business (GMB)

Search Engine Optimization (SEO)

Surgical Care Affiliates

https://scasurgery.com/

United Surgical Partners International

https://www.uspi.com/

Amsurg

https://www.amsurg.com/

Surgical Center Development

http://www.surgcenter.com/

About the Author

Kevin Kruse M.D. is a board-certified orthopedic surgeon with fellowship training in the shoulder, elbow, and hand. Dr. Kruse obtained his undergraduate and medical degrees from Indiana University. While in college, he played linebacker for the Indiana Hoosiers' football team and earned Academic All-Big Ten honors. He credits his experience of playing football in high school and college with teaching him valuable life lessons including working as a team, developing discipline, and dealing with failure. His participation in football set the foundation for his work ethic and approach to success.

Dr. Kruse completed his Orthopedic Surgery residency at Greenville Health System University Medical Center in Greenville, South Carolina, where he trained with the Steadman Hawkins Clinic of the Carolinas. Next, he went on to complete a hand and upper extremity fellowship at the University of Pittsburgh Medical Center, before traveling to Lyon, France to complete a four-month fellowship in shoulder surgery at the Centre Orthopedique Santy with world-renowned shoulder surgeon, Gilles Walch. Dr. Kruse believes that the opportunity for him (and his young family) to immerse themselves in French culture and to learn specialized shoulder surgery in another country opened his mind and shaped the surgical practice he manages today more than any other part of his training.

The publisher of several papers on shoulder, elbow, and hand surgery, Dr. Kruse has presented at medical meetings throughout the United States. His research interests include management of rotator cuff tears, shoulder arthroplasty, and the use of ultrasound in the shoulder. He is a member of the Arthroscopy Association of North America, American Society for Surgery of the Hand, (ASSH) and American Shoulder and Elbow Surgeons (ASES).

After relocating to Dallas with his wife Stephanie (a former Indianapolis Colts cheerleader) and his children, Dr. Kruse accepted a job with a busy orthopedic group, where he put his "Dr. Hustle" philosophy into practice. His application of 9 core principles resulted in the establishment of a thriving, successful practice in one of the country's most competitive environments.

When not working, he enjoys spending time with Stephanie and their three children Livia, Violet, and Kace; cooking; golfing; reading; and weightlifting.

Acknowledgements

Dr. Joseph Imbriglia

Dr. Richard Hawkins

Dr. Gilles Walch

Dr. Mark Baratz

Dr. Chris Schmidt

Dr. Dean Sotereanos

Dr. Kyle Jeray

Dr. John Millon

Dr. John Leonard Sanders

Dr. Michael Kissenberth

Dr. Ed Rudisill

Dr. Bob Scheinburg

Dr. Brett Raynor